"The authors offer an excellent discussion of PMDD that is understandable and chock-full of sound information. I heartily recommend this book to women who suffer from PMDD and their health professionals, as well as to their family and friends who would like a more extensive knowledge of the problem."

—Karen L. Salley, Ph.D., Professor of Psychology and Women's Studies, Southern Oregon University

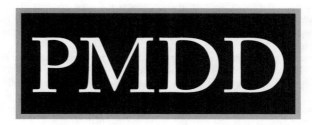

PMDD

A GUIDE TO COPING WITH
Premenstrual Dysphoric Disorder

James E. Huston, M.D. &
Lani C. Fujitsubo, Ph.D.

New Harbinger Publications, Inc.

Publisher's Note

Distributed in the U.S.A. by Publishers Group West; in Canada by Raincoast Books; in Great Britain by Airlift Book Company, Ltd.; in South Africa by Real Books, Ltd.; in Australia by Boobook; and in New Zealand by Tandem Press.

Copyright © 2002 by James E. Huston and Lani C. Fujitsubo
New Harbinger Publications, Inc.
5674 Shattuck Avenue
Oakland, CA 94609

Pages 17–18, 119–121, and 125 reprinted with permission from the *Diagnostic and Statistical Manual of Mental Disorders, Fourth Edition, Text Revision.* Copyright 2000 American Psychiatric Association.

Cover design by Amy Shoup
Cover image by Geoff du Feu/Getty Images
Edited by Brady Kahn
Text design by Michele Waters

ISBN 1-57224-283-3 Paperback

All Rights Reserved

Printed in the United States of America

New Harbinger Publications' Web site address: www.newharbinger.com

04   03   02

10   9   8   7   6   5   4   3   2   1

First printing

Contents

OCT   2002

PART 4
Overview

Preface

Much, yet not enough, is known about premenstrual dysphoric disorder (PMDD), the chaos that engulfs millions of women on a monthly basis, disrupting the daily functioning of their lives and the lives of those around them. PMDD is a severe form of premenstrual syndrome (PMS). For centuries, it has been recognized that women are susceptible to mood and bodily changes just before their menstrual periods are due. Until fairly recently, though, these troublesome changes were dismissed as merely a part of feminity: "Women do this sort of thing. Get used to it," was the typical attitude.

Social and scientific interest in these premenstrual changes has evolved over the past few decades. But so far medical researchers have not been able to find a sole, underlying cause for PMDD, or consequently, a sole cure. Rather, many adverse influences appear to underlie this condition. Hundreds of publications reporting on scientific studies have expressed myriad opinions and observations about premenstrual changes. Of the available information on PMDD, some is based on good science, some on pseudo-science, some on personal belief, and some on little more than myth. Advocates of different schools of thought abound.

In spite of this, good information is available, and help exists. There is no reason to continue to suffer from the cyclic chaos of PMDD simply because neither you nor your health advisors are well enough informed. Our purpose in writing this book is to gather the most reliable information from a mountain of published data, and present a comprehensive guide for identifying, understanding, and dealing with PMDD.

One further note: Some members of the medical community and others continue to doubt whether PMDD should be regarded as a medical condition. We hope to dispel these doubts, and help eliminate the negative image that a diagnosis of PMDD often confers on women who suffer from it.

Ongoing research will continue to reveal additional fundamental facts about PMDD. Meanwhile, there is information available to help you and millions of other women cope successfully with premenstrual dysphoric disorder. We present it in this book.

James E. Huston, M.D.
Lani C. Fujitsubo, Ph.D.

Foreword

For many women, life takes on a bumpy course of shifting energy, chaotic feelings, and physical discomfort as they move through their monthly menstrual cycle. For about five percent of women, the ten days before menstruation become a tortuous and out-of-control experience that wreak havoc on their internal well-being as well as on loved ones, friends, and work. These women may be suffering from premenstrual dysphoric disorder (PMDD), a devastating condition that affects every aspect of life. Although PMDD has probably always been here, it has only recently become recognized and treated as a genuine disorder by the medical establishment.

This book is for women who want to understand and take control of their adverse experience, and for the health providers who want to help them. With frankness, thoroughness, and humor, Huston and Fujitsubo explain the multiple physical causes of PMDD, the environmental factors that make matters worse, and the broad range of specific approaches that can help. They complete these tasks with a deep commitment to validate PMDD and the women who experience it. They debunk myths and elaborate every currently known treatment. Their attitude is holistic and inclusive, embracing not only conventional medicine but also the importance of nutrition, exercise, and stress management, as well as possible roles for psychotherapy and alternative medicine. The authors empower women with information and specific guidelines for how to evaluate PMDD and how to implement various interventions.

I commend Huston and Fujitsubo for the breadth, depth, and accessibility of their work. This is a book with answers for women who want to get back in control again, so that life is exhilarating and enriching, a celebration with lots of room for happiness and joy, every day of the month.

Josie A. Wilson, Ph.D.
Chair Department of Psychology
Southern Oregon University

The Nature of Premenstrual Dysphoric Disorder

In addressing what it's like to undergo the turmoil of premenstrual symptoms, Academy Award nominee Janet McTeer put it well in the movie *Tumbleweeds*: "It isn't easy being female. Just ask any woman right before Aunt Rose pays her monthly visit." She knew, didn't she? Most women have experienced that irritable, aching, bloated, anxious feeling, but few know why it happens. In part I, we will describe what happens to your body when you have PMDD and discuss the disorder's extent in the population; who is at risk; and how PMDD is recognized. We will show you that premenstrual dysphoric disorder is a true bodily condition that arises from biologic changes over which you have little control. PMDD is not mental illness. We will present the science to prove this to you. Armed with this background information, you will more readily understand the balance of the book which is devoted to relieving PMDD.

CHAPTER 1

What Is PMDD and Who Gets It?

Symptoms and bodily changes associated with the menstrual cycle have been recognized and described for centuries, so we are not talking about anything new here. This chapter will briefly review how the menstrual cycle works and will examine premenstrual dysphoric disorder and how it differs from premenstrual syndrome. You will see that they are actually variations of the same condition, the difference being one of degree. We will show you how medical knowledge about premenstrual symptoms has evolved mostly in the past seventy years, the bulk of it during the past three decades. Finally, we will explain the scope of the problem posed by PMDD for millions of women, which points up the need for broader understanding among women, among those with whom they have relationships, and among their health advisors.

How Does the Menstrual Cycle Work?

The Reproductive Organs

The uterus is a pear-shaped organ about the size of your fist located in the pelvis between your bladder and lower intestine. It consists of two parts: the body and the cervix. Pregnancies implant themselves in the body, which expands as the baby grows. The lower one-third, the cervix, has a canal opening into the vagina, which is the exit passage for menstrual flow. Leading off each side of the uterine body are the two fallopian tubes. Each tube ends in the vicinity of an ovary. Ovaries contain the egg cells, which initiate a new life when contact is made with a male sperm cell. The fertilized egg cell is transported to the uterus through a fallopian tube.

The inner lining of the uterus is called the endometrium. In the second half of the menstrual cycle, called the luteal phase, it becomes thickened and enriched with blood vessels and the glands become engorged with glycogen, a sugar, for nourishment of the tiny embryo. If a pregnancy does not occur, the endometrium is shed as part of the menstrual flow.

The Reproductive Hormone Cycle

The cycle is really sort of a daisy chain, as you can see in figure 1.1. The chain involves three hormone-producing glands:

- the hypothalamus, in the brain

- the pituitary, in the brain

- the ovaries, in the pelvis

These glands work in concert with each other. Each produces hormones that are recognized by the other two, acting as chemical messengers that are carried to their targets by your bloodstream. Some of these hormones influence the ovarian cycle.

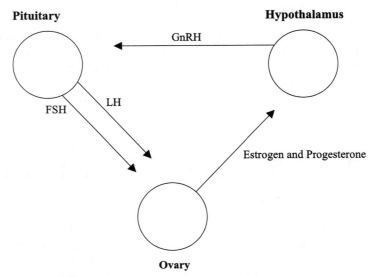

Figure 1.1 Ovarian Cycle

We need to start our discussion somewhere in the cycle, so let's enter it at the end of a menstrual period, after the uterine lining has been shed. At this point, your ovaries are producing low levels of estrogen and progesterone, as figure 1.2 demonstrates. This is called the follicular phase of the cycle. The hypothalamus detects this and sends a hormone called gonadotropin releasing hormone (GnRH) to the pituitary. In response, the pituitary releases two hormones that target the ovaries: follicle stimulating hormone (FSH) and leuteinizing hormone (LH). FSH stimulates the ovaries to do two things: start producing more estrogen (which, among other things, rebuilds the lining of the uterus) and get some follicles ready for ovulation. At mid-cycle, estrogen reaches a critical level, which triggers a sudden surge of LH from the pituitary; this causes ovulation. Now the luteal phase of the cycle begins.

After the follicle has released its egg, it turns into a structure called the *corpus luteum*, which manufactures progesterone. Progesterone increases the blood supply in the uterine lining and fills the glands of the lining with glycogen (a sugar). This prepares the lining of the uterus for receiving and nourishing a fertilized egg.

At this point the bloodstream contains high levels of estrogen and progesterone. If conception has not occurred, the hypothalamus reduces the GnRH level, signaling the pituitary to cut back on FSH and LH. This in turn causes the ovaries to decrease estrogen and progesterone production. The net result is that, once again, the bloodstream contains a low level of female hormones. The lining of the uterus is no longer supported by hormones, and it is shed—in other words, a menstrual period occurs. Then the cycle, which usually takes about four weeks, begins again.

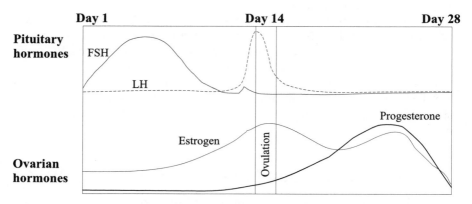

Figure 1.2   Hormone Levels in Menstrual Cycle

What Is Premenstrual Dysphoric Disorder?

A person exhibiting dysphoria is someone with excessive pain, anguish, or agitation. It is derived from the Greek word *dusphoros*, which means hard to bear.

Premenstrual Syndrome (PMS)

To more clearly understand premenstrual dysphoric disorder (PMDD), it will be helpful to first define premenstrual syndrome. PMS is no longer considered a single condition, but rather a group of disorders and symptoms related to the menstrual cycle. It is a complex psychological-neurological-hormonal disorder represented by a variable collection of physical, emotional, and behavioral symptoms arising in the late luteal phase (seven to ten days before the menstrual period), and which are known to affect a woman's physical and emotional well-being (Mortola 1994). The symptoms vary from cycle to cycle and from woman to woman, and disappear after the onset of menstrual flow. More than 100 physical and psychological symptoms are recognized, including irritability, mild to moderate mood disturbances, bloating, abdominal pain, weight gain, increased appetite with food cravings, sore breasts, and headache (Pearlstein and Stone 1998; Frye and Silverman 2000). PMS doesn't affect every woman, but 85 to 90 percent of women experience at least some of the symptoms, although not of sufficient magnitude to require medical or psychological interventions (Parker 1994). Up to 40 percent of women of reproductive age experience premenstrual symptoms that qualify for a diagnosis of PMS (Woods et al. 1986).

Several organizations have developed diagnostic criteria for PMS including the World Health Organization (1996) and the American College of Obstetricians and Gynecologists (ACOG 2000). The *International Classification of Diseases* (ICD-10), published by the WHO, stresses that in PMS, physical symptoms predominate over psychological ones. PMS differs from PMDD in that no minimum number of symptoms must be present to establish a diagnosis (Steiner 1996). We will cover this further later in the chapter.

Premenstrual Dysphoric Disorder (PMDD)

PMDD is a severe variant, or subset, of PMS mood disorders, and not an independent condition. PMDD symptoms go far beyond what are considered manageable or usual symptoms. PMDD is characterized by mood disorders of sufficient magnitude to interfere with social or occupational relationships, or vocational functioning. The *physical* symptoms of PMDD are similar to PMS; it is the severe mood changes that constitute the difference. They may include irritability, anxiety, depressed mood, insomnia, diminished self-image, emotional hypersensitivity, poor concentration, angry outbursts, lack of control, and more (see table 1.1).

Historical Review

Hippocrates, the ancient Greek physician of "Hippocratic Oath" fame, wrote about menstrual disorders for the first time in recorded history. He coined the term *hysteria*, which he thought was caused by the uterus wandering throughout the body wreaking havoc wherever it went. Interesting idea, but dead wrong.

Premenstrual symptomatology has been acknowledged for centuries. In 1847, Dr. Ernst F. von Feuchtersleben wrote: "The menses in sensitive women is almost always attended by mental uneasiness, irritability, and sadness." Ernst was onto something.

In the twentieth century, Robert Frank, an American obstetrician/ gynecologist, published a paper in 1931 on *premenstrual tension*. That term was widely used until Katharina Dalton, a British obstetrician/gynecologist, coined the term *premenstrual syndrome*, and received worldwide acclaim for more accurately describing the condition. Dalton reasoned that PMS was caused by a deficiency in progesterone, the dominant female hormone in the second half of the menstrual cycle. She was wrong, but her beliefs and writings resulted in women using tons of progesterone vaginal suppositories to treat PMS for most of two decades. It was eventually shown that progesterone treatment for PMS was no more effective than a placebo. But Dalton put PMS on the map, and her work stimulated hundreds of studies.

The psychiatric community got involved in the 1980s because PMS was so suggestive of a mental disorder with its mood swings, loss of emotional control, fits of anger, and more. The result of psychiatric interest was that in 1987, PMS was renamed *late luteal phase dysphoric disorder* (LLPDD). The American Psychiatric Association (APA) was not convinced that LLPDD was a mental illness, however, so rather than list it in the main text, it was included in the appendix of the *Diagnostic and Statistical Manual of Mental Disorders* (*DSM-III*). After further studies, the APA concluded that women who have premenstrual symptoms are not necessarily mentally ill. This led to renaming the condition *premenstrual dysphoric disorder* (PMDD) in the *DSM-IV* (1994), and the recognition that the disorder is one of mood. Because PMDD can be differentiated from the milder PMS, *DSM-IV* guidelines were developed to establish diagnostic criteria for PMDD. (These are covered in chapter 2.)

Table 1.1
Symptoms of Premenstrual Dysphoric Disorder

Psychological
Irritability, Agitation
Lack of control
Easily overwhelmed
Emotional hypersensitivity
Anxiety, Nervousness
Anger, Rage, Hostility
Poor concentration
Confusion, Forgetfulness
Decision difficulty
Sadness, Depression
Lethargy, Severe fatigue
Insomnia
Wanting to be alone
Diminished self-image
Tearfulness
Moodiness

Neurological and
 Vascular
Headache
Dizziness
Fainting
Numbness, tingling in arms
   and/or legs
Heart palpitations
Easy bruising
Muscle spasms

Fluid retention
Cyclic weight gain
Edema—ankles, feet, hands
Breast fullness and pain
Decreased urine output

Skin problems
Acne
Aggravation of cold sores or
   other skin conditions
Neurodermatitis (itching and
   inflammation)

Gastrointestinal
Bloating
Nausea
Vomiting
Abdominal cramps
Constipation
Pelvic heaviness

Respiratory
Infections
Allergies

Eye complaints
Conjunctivitis
Visual disturbances

Other changes
Food cravings
Decreased sexual desire
Increased sexual desire
Hot flashes
Menstrual cramps
Clumsiness

Adapted from: Premenstrual Dysphoric Disorder; www.baptistoneword.org;
May 10, 2001

So, that's how PMDD has evolved. In recent years, the term has acquired a certain cachet; PMDD is the term of preference for people publishing articles in the medical literature or on the Internet. Chat rooms have evolved, which have propagated myths and propaganda. But the bottom line is, PMDD is PMS, although it is a ferocious form of PMS due to its serious mood disorders.

Scope of the Problem

One in twenty (up to 5 percent) of approximately 70 million American women in the childbearing age group meets the diagnostic criteria for PMDD (as discussed in chapter 2). Some quote this figure as between 3 and 9 percent. This means up to 3 to 5 million women undergo these severe cyclic mood changes on a regular monthly basis. In spite of this large number of affected women, a recent survey of 500 women commissioned by the Society for the Advancement of Women's Health Research found a low awareness of the term *premenstrual dysphoric disorder* (Women's Health Research 1999). Indeed, only 16 percent of respondents had ever heard of PMDD. Among women with severe premenstrual symptoms, more than one quarter (27 percent) had never even discussed their symptoms with their doctors. This was in spite of the fact that their symptoms were interfering with their daily lives, especially relationships with family and friends. Ninety percent preferred to cope on their own because seeking help was regarded as a sign of weakness. About one-quarter felt their complaints would not be taken seriously by their doctor, or they might become the butt of jokes. That's a sad commentary on how well we have educated American women and American health advisors about this disorder.

Women who seek help and advice for PMDD and PMS basically want to be validated. They want to be assured that they have a physiologic disorder, and not a psychiatric illness. Some researchers are concerned that the inclusion of PMDD in the psychiatric diagnostic literature, such as *DSM-IV*, may misrepresent the problem. Women who suffer from PMDD and their physicians may come to view the condition only as a psychiatric disorder and not as a condition with biologic causes unrelated to mental disorders. The worry is that categorizing PMDD as a psychiatric disorder may restrict research exclusively to psychiatric areas.

An additional problem is that spouses, children, family members, friends, neighbors, coworkers, bosses, and clients interface daily with PMDD sufferers. The chronic monthly dysfunction of PMDD is well known to have an adverse influence on interpersonal relationships, occupational associates, and vocational achievement. This broadens the scope of the problem considerably, given that women tend to define themselves through their relationships with other people, and suffer much more than men when a relationship has gone awry. Men tend to place higher core value on physical ability, occupational success, sexual prowess, and societal impact. But women feel most secure when relationships are intact and stable, so a relationship glitch is a significant disruption (Kaplan 1986). PMDD also magnifies depression and other mood disorders, and may even result in some women entertaining suicidal as well as homicidal thoughts (APA 1994).

So, PMDD is not only extremely unsettling to the women who experience it, but the consequences of the disorder may have negative effects on other people important to their lives. Thus, the case is well made for giving PMDD the serious consideration that a significant disorder deserves, and for educating women and the general public, as well as health care advisors, more broadly about the nuances of this condition.

CHAPTER 2

Medical Information: What's Known, What Isn't

As a result of more widespread study in the past thirty years, and especially in the past ten years, much more information has emerged on PMDD. This chapter will go into detail on the incidence and symptoms of PMDD, what is known about the cause or causes, who is at risk, and the criteria for establishing a diagnosis.

Incidence

PMDD and PMS occur only during the childbearing years. Women who do not have functioning ovaries do not have PMDD or PMS. Although it can start in the teens, the age range for most women is from the mid- to late-twenties until menopause in the early fifties. Women who seek treatment are usually in their thirties (Yonkers 1997). It is common for symptoms to worsen in the perimenopausal years, from roughly age thirty-five to fifty (Huston and Lanka 2001). Some women are completely free of PMS or PMDD until they experience its onset in their mid-forties. Members of this latter group often benefit from female hormone supplements. (More on this in chapter 6.)

As mentioned earlier, 85 to 90 percent of women experience some symptoms of PMS, but only about 40 percent of those meet the criteria for a diagnosis. Still fewer (3 to 9 percent) meet the criteria for PMDD (Yonkers 1997).

Causes of PMDD

In the past, several theories have been advanced as to the cause or causes of PMDD, including that it may be a stress-induced disorder, a variant of a mood disorder, or a personality disorder. The compelling evidence, however, is that none of these psychologically based theories can fully explain what causes PMDD. It is known that PMDD can be distinguished from a mood disorder both biochemically and by psychometric tests (Mortola 1995). Thus, it isn't surprising that treatment based solely on psychological intervention fails to provide complete relief for full-blown PMDD.

PMDD symptoms occur when your brain is unable to maintain its usual chemical balance during the one to two weeks prior to your menstrual period. Shortly after the onset of menstrual flow, your brain reestablishes the balance, and symptoms disappear.

Although no single cause has been confirmed, the fact that PMDD coincides with the menstrual cycle has led researchers to believe that normal ovarian functioning (rather than female hormone imbalance) is the cyclical trigger for PMDD-related events within the central nervous system and other target organs (Steiner 2000). In other words, if you have PMDD, you have an underlying neurobiological vulnerability, or abnormal biochemical response, to your own normal fluctuations in circulating female hormones. Both women who suffer from PMDD and those who are unaffected undergo the same cyclic hormonal changes. What differs is how the central nervous system responds to those changes. (Schmidt, Nieman, and Danaceau 1998). Hormones and chemicals from all over the body are implicated. They include:

- **ovarian hormones:** estrogen and progesterone

- **pituitary hormones:** follicle stimulating hormone (FSH), luteinizing hormone (LH), and prolactin

- **endorphins:** opium-like chemicals produced in the midbrain and hypothalamus

- **neurotransmitters:** serotonin, gamma-aminobutyric acid (GABA), dopamine, and norepinephrine

- **adrenal hormone:** cortisol

So, PMDD is a hormone and brain-biochemistry problem that results in mood and behavioral derangements. In many ways it's a relief for women to realize that it is a recognized medical condition with biological roots and not a mental illness.

The symptoms originate in two areas of the brain known as the *limbic* area and the *cerebral cortex*. The above neurotransmitters connect these two areas, and any change in the level of these chemicals can affect a woman's mood and daily functioning (British Columbia Reproductive Mental

Health Program 2001). These brain areas control some very important functions. The limbic area controls memory, sleep, appetite, and strong emotions such as anger, rage, and aggression. The cerebral cortex controls concentration, attention, judgment, moods, perceptions, views, and interpretations of what is happening to you and around you.

Although PMDD remains poorly understood, symptoms are thought to come from an altered sensitivity to neurotransmitters (Kessel 2000). What *is* known, however, is that women suffering from PMDD have serotonin dysregulation resulting in low levels in the late luteal phase of their cycle. Serotonin has been shown to be the main player in causing PMS and PMDD. This discovery has finally pinned down a chemical cause for PMDD, and led the way to a treatment that works.

Serotonin is one of your body's "feel good" chemicals. It is produced by nerve cells, called neurons, and its function as a neurotransmitter is to facilitate the transmission of nerve impulses from one neuron to the next. When impulse transmission is occurring, serotonin is released by the involved neurons; and, while it is outside the neuron, serotonin produces a calming effect. However, neurons can also recapture the released serotonin, and when they do so in large enough amounts, a low serotonin level results, which in PMDD results in depressed mood, irritability, anger, aggression, poor control of impulses, and carbohydrate cravings (Eriksson 1999). This observation led to the use of drugs that prevent the reuptake of serotonin by nerve cells, called *selective serotonin reuptake inhibitors* (SSRIs). (More on this in chapter 6.)

Norepinephrine, also a neurotransmitter, is a brain chemical that plays a very important role in regulating mood. Abnormal levels of this chemical have been strongly implicated in depression. It has now been documented that abnormally high levels of norepinephrine and abnormally low levels of *cortisol* are present in people subjected to chronic stress. Since PMDD is often associated with chronic stress, it may be that norepinephrine plays an important role in causing it (Girdler et al. 1998).

Gamma-aminobutyric acid (GABA) is an inhibitory neurotransmitter that suppresses the firing of nerve cells, thus preventing excessive brain stimulation. In the follicular phase of the cycle GABA levels are the same in women with PMDD as in nonaffected women, but in the luteal phase (when PMDD occurs), GABA levels fail to rise as they do in women who do not have PMDD (Pearlstein and Stone 1998). As a result, overstimulation of brain cells occurs.

Allopregnanolone is another chemical that is being studied for its role in PMDD. It is a *metabolite* (breakdown product) of progesterone, the female sex hormone, and is known to be neuroactive. Allopregnanolone is a GABA agonist, meaning it enhances the inhibitory effect of GABA. A University of North Carolina study reported by Dr. Susan Girdler showed that allopregnanolone levels rise during stress in normal women, suggesting it helps control stress responses (Girdler et al. 2001). In women with

PMDD the levels are higher than they are in nonaffected women, but in times of stress, their allopregnanolone levels do not rise nearly as well. Women with the most severe PMDD symptoms had lower levels of allopregnanolone than the less symptomatic PMDD women. This suggests that dysregulation of allopregnanolone mechanisms occurs in PMDD, and that further investigation is warranted. Low levels of both GABA and allopregnanolone diminishes their protective effect on the brain and this is thought to allow the appearance of premenstrual mood symptoms.

Calcium deficiency is also being intensely studied as a possible contributor to PMDD. It has been found that 1,200 milligrams of calcium per day reduces symptoms for about half the women who have PMDD. This observation has convinced Dr. Susan Thys-Jacobs that PMDD is not a mental illness (Thys-Jacobs et al. 1998). She feels that PMDD/PMS symptoms are the body's way of informing you on a monthly basis that you have a calcium deficiency.

Beta-endorphins are opium-like brain chemicals that are your body's natural painkilling hormones. Women with PMDD have been shown to have lower than normal levels of beta-endorphins, and a decreased tolerance for pain (Girdler 2000). The unusual aspect of this finding is that low beta-endorphin levels are present *continuously* in women with PMDD, not just premenstrually. Women with PMDD are more sensitive to pain. This finding supports a growing body of evidence suggesting that PMDD is a chronic disorder that causes abnormal levels of many hormones on a continuous basis throughout the month.

Prolactin is a pituitary hormone involved in breast milk production. Premenstrual breast tenderness has been shown by Turkish investigators to be associated with increased levels of this hormone (Kaleli et al. 2001). When women were treated with lisuride maleate, a prolactin-lowering drug, the hormone levels dropped and breast tenderness decreased significantly.

So far, the information collected on PMDD is a piecemeal assembly by a large number of investigators. The full picture has not yet been completed.

PMDD Look-alikes

Because PMDD/PMS can mimic a number of mood and behavior disorders as well as medical conditions, it's essential to get an accurate diagnosis before you decide on an appropriate therapy. Three areas are easily confused with PMDD/PMS and must be kept in mind when PMDD/PMS is being considered as a diagnosis.

1. **Premenstrual magnification of an underlying mood disorder.** Mood disorders such as major depression, dysthymia (prolonged

mild depression), anxiety disorder, bipolar disorder, and panic disorder are commonly exaggerated premenstrually. Up to 50 percent of women incorrectly diagnosed with PMDD/PMS will be found to have an underlying mood disorder (Mortola 1997). Fatigue, pain, and other manifestations similar to premenstrual symptoms may also be produced by an underactive thyroid (hypothyroidism) and other chronic medical conditions such as diabetes, anemia, lupus and other autoimmune disorders, fibrocystic breasts, chronic fatigue syndrome, irritable bowel syndrome, asthma, seizure disorders, migraine headaches, and endometriosis (ACOG 2000).

2. **Perimenopausal symptoms.** After age forty, estrogen production begins to fluctuate in many women to a degree that results in moodiness, loss of concentration, and fatigue resembling PMDD/PMS.

3. **Oral contraceptives.** Mood alterations that can occur may be confused with PMDD/PMS.

The bottom line here is that PMDD and PMS are diagnoses of exclusion. If you can eliminate the above psychological and physical problems as diagnostic possibilities, you will be on firmer ground in considering PMDD/PMS as the source of your premenstrual symptoms.

Risk Factors for PMDD

Premenstrual symptoms are reported in all cultures worldwide. While any woman with functioning ovaries can develop PMDD, certain other factors can increase the risk:

1. **Family history of PMS or PMDD.** This is especially the case if it is your mother or sister (ACOG 2000). Studies of identical twins with PMDD show a 93 percent chance of both having the disorder compared to 44 percent in fraternal twins and 31 percent in sisters who were not twins (Condon 1993). Researchers are looking for the underlying genetic process.

2. **Personal or family history of depression.** Forty percent of women with PMDD have a history of major depression either personally or in their family (Bailey and Cohen 1999).

3. **Personal or family history of mood disorders.** These include panic attacks, bipolar disorder (formerly manic-depressive disorder), anxiety disorder, and seasonal affective disorder (SAD). Austrian researchers found that 46 percent of women with SAD (a cyclic depressive condition seen in winter) also met the diagnostic criteria for PMDD (Praschak-Rieder et al. 2001).

4. **Personal or family history of postpartum depression.** The brain is thought to have an imprint of this experience, which it incorporates into its mood and anxiety pathways. This paves the way for adverse emotional, physical, and behavioral responses to cyclic hormonal changes.

5. **Childhood sexual or physical abuse.** More than half of women with PMDD have histories of physical or sexual abuse during childhood or adolescence (Girdler et al. 1998). The expected incidence of this type of abuse in the general population of women is 20 to 25 percent.

6. **Chronic exposure to stress.** In women with chronic, ongoing stress in their lives, stress hormones are continuously maintained at abnormal levels: norepinephrine is too high and cortisol is too low. PMDD is much more likely in such women, suggesting that it is related to dysregulation of the stress response (Girdler et al. 1998).

7. PMDD is associated with, but not proven to be caused by:
   - a lower education level
   - current cigarette smoking
   - small children at home
   - working outside the home
   - eating disorders
   - sedentary lifestyle

Diagnosis

There are no routine laboratory tests or physical examination techniques that are useful in determining whether you do or do not have PMDD. The diagnosis must be based on your accurately reporting what actually happens to you. Even though you may be quite uncomfortable premenstrually, with headaches, cramps, breast tenderness, and moodiness, this is not necessarily premenstrual dysphoric disorder (Yonkers 1999). To be considered PMDD, these physical symptoms must be accompanied by cyclical mood and behavioral changes of such severity that they cause marked impairment in your ability to function in day-to-day interactions in your various relationships at home, at work, at school, or other social encounters. Signs of psychosocial impairment include marital discord, parenting difficulties, poor work performance, and increasing social isolation (Mortola 1992). Psychosocial impairments alone do not constitute PMDD, however, unless you also undergo cyclical mood changes.

The DSM-IV Definition

The *Diagnostic and Statistical Manual of Mental Disorders* (*DSM-IV*) is quite specific in its delineation (APA 1994). A diagnosis of PMDD requires at least five symptoms that coincide with functional impairment during most cycles of the past year. PMS differs from PMDD in that no minimum number of symptoms is required nor is functional impairment required for a PMS diagnosis.

The strict *DSM-IV* requirements for PMDD are as follows:

A. In most menstrual cycles during the past year, five (or more) of the following symptoms were present for most of the time during the last week of the luteal phase, began to remit within a few days after the onset of the menstrual flow and were absent in the week postmenses, with at least one of the five symptoms being either (1), (2), (3), or (4):

   1. markedly depressed mood, feelings of hopelessness, or self-deprecating thoughts
   2. marked anxiety, tension, feelings of being "keyed up," or "on edge"
   3. marked affective lability (e.g., feeling suddenly sad or tearful or increased sensitivity to rejection)
   4. persistent and marked anger or irritability or increased interpersonal conflicts
   5. decreased interest in usual activities (e.g., work, school, friends, hobbies)
   6. subjective sense of difficulty in concentrating
   7. lethargy, easy fatigability, or marked lack of energy
   8. marked change in appetite, overeating, or specific food cravings
   9. hypersomnia or insomnia
   10. a subjective sense of being overwhelmed or out of control
   11. other physical symptoms, such as breast tenderness or swelling, headaches, joint or muscle pain, a sensation of "bloating," weight gain

B. The disturbance markedly interferes with work or school or with usual social activities and relationships with others (e.g., avoidance of social activities, decreased productivity and efficiency at work or school).

C. The disturbance is not merely an exacerbation of the symptoms of another disorder, such as major depression disorder, panic disorder, dysthymia disorder or a personality disorder (although it may be superimposed on any of these disorders).

D. Criteria A, B, and C must be confirmed by prospective daily rat-ings during at least two consecutive symptomatic cycles. (717-718)

Those are pretty strict criteria, but other researchers found that two more factors should be taken into account (Steiner, Steinberg, and Stewart 1995):

1. If your symptoms don't abate by the end of menstruation, you don't have PMDD or PMS. There must be a symptom-free interval during the follicular phase (the first half) of your cycle.

2. For you to be diagnosed with PMDD your symptoms within any given cycle must grow worse by at least 30 percent from the follicular phase to the luteal phase (second half). These researchers suggest that your symptoms must grow worse by at least 50 per-cent to merit drug treatment.

Some people are beginning to feel that the criteria for diagnosing PMDD may be too stringent. It is entirely possible for some women to experience noticeable difficulty with premenstrual functioning in one or another sphere of their lives yet not meet the diagnostic criteria for PMDD. These women may be denied needed treatment. This issue requires further debate and research.

Rating Your Symptoms

To evaluate the worsening, or improving, of premenstrual symptoms some researchers have developed scoring systems. Here are two of the more prominent ones that you might find useful:

1. **Prospective Record of the Impact and Severity of Menstruation (PRISM).** This asks you to rate each of your symptoms for severity using a range of 0, for no impact, to 7, for severe impact (Reid 1985).

2. **Calendar of Premenstrual Experiences (COPE).** The range for this scoring system is 0 to 3 (Mortola et al. 1990).

It doesn't matter which of these two scoring methods you use. Each represents nothing more than a simple system to rate your PMDD symptoms.

Keeping a Diary

Keeping a diary to record your symptoms is a necessary step in determining if you have PMDD or PMS. You should keep it for at least two consecutive months during which you have symptoms and then review the results with your doctor. Use an ordinary calendar:

1. Mark the first day of your menstrual flow as "Day 1."

2. Count forward twenty-eight days (or the average length of your cycle) and mark that date as the expected date of your next menstrual period.

3. From that date, count back 10 days and mark the date that you expect your premenstrual symptoms to begin.

4. Throughout the entire month, not just the last ten days, record your symptoms from the eleven categories in the *DSM-IV* listing above. You can save time and space by recording only the number of the appropriate category. If you are rating the severity of your symptoms, put the PRISM or COPE score in parenthesis beside the number.

5. It's also helpful to keep a journal for recording additional symptoms not covered in the list of eleven.

There are several advantages in your keeping a symptom diary. First, your symptom ratings will show the pattern in which they occur, confirming or refuting your impression of what has been happening to you over months or years. Your diary will also serve as a visual aid, which will make it easier for you and your health advisor to decide whether or not your pattern is consistent with PMDD/PMS. Finally, by charting and rating your symptoms, you may gain a sense of control over them. Visualizing the type, severity, and timing of your symptoms can make them seem more manageable. For many women, this sense of control is actually enough to relieve some of the distress they feel and make other management interventions unnecessary.

Your completion of a daily symptom diary over two menstrual cycles, will reveal the major symptoms that bother you, as well as their pattern of appearance. This information can be quite valuable during subsequent efforts to deal with your condition and evaluate your improvement. (Self-help and medical interventions are covered in parts 2 and 3). From the diary, it will also be possible to establish which of the following five diagnostic categories applies to you (Steiner and Wilkins 1996).

1. **PMDD:** This means you meet the *DSM-IV* criteria, and have no other ongoing psychiatric disorder. Your diary shows you have one of the four core symptoms and at least five of the eleven total symptom categories. You can state that they have occurred with

most of your cycles for the past year, and have been severe enough to have interfered in the daily functioning of your social and occupational roles. Your symptoms demonstrate clear worsening premenstrually, and they stop within a few days of menstrual flow onset. If your symptoms have worsened by 50 percent from the follicular phase to the luteal phase, you merit drug intervention.

2. **PMS:** You do not meet the *DSM-IV* criteria for PMDD, but do meet the *ICD-10* criteria for premenstrual syndrome (World Health Organization 1987). These include mild psychological discomfort and feelings of bloating, temporary weight gain, breast tenderness and swelling, various aches and pains, poor concentration, sleep disturbance, change in appetite, swelling of hands and feet. Only one of these symptoms is required for a PMS diagnosis. It must occur in the premenstrual phase of your cycle, reach a peak shortly before menstruation, and cease with the onset of flow or shortly thereafter.

3. **Premenstrual Magnification:** This refers to a situation in which you meet the criteria for either PMDD or PMS, but also have a current major psychiatric disorder (major depression, bipolar disorder, panic attacks, anxiety disorder), or you have another unstable medical condition (thyroid disease, irritable bowel, lupus, endometriosis, fibromyalgia, menstrual migraine). All of these conditions can be magnified in severity premenstrually, and many of them mimic PMS or PMDD symptoms. The difference is that with another concurrent condition (e.g., major depression), you do not become symptom-free after the onset of menstrual flow. You have symptoms all the time, but they get worse premenstrually. (See figure 2.1.)

4. **Other Psychiatric Diagnosis:** You do not have symptoms that meet the criteria for either PMS or PMDD, but some of your symptoms meet the *DSM-IV* criteria for another psychiatric disorder. It is quite common for major depression to be revealed this way. Cyclical mental illnesses such as intermittent depressive disorder and cyclothymia may fall into this category; cycles for these disorders do not correspond to the menstrual cycle.

5. **No Diagnosis:** You may have premenstrual symptoms, some of which may be disruptive, but they are not severe enough to warrant a diagnosis of PMDD or PMS.

Deciding which category best applies to you will help you design the management interventions most suitable for your individual situation. For example, if you are found to have PMDD with premenstrual magnification of coexisting depression, it may be prudent to treat the depression first as the more threatening of the two. If "no diagnosis" is your result, and

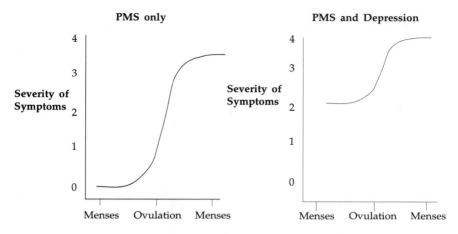

Figure 2.1.   Premenstrual Syndrome with Depression

chronic stress is found to be the cause of your symptoms, then conservative measures such as diet and lifestyle changes or group psychotherapy may be the best measures for you. As you will see later in the book, no single therapy relieves all the symptoms of PMDD. Successful management involves a regimen of interventions tailored for your needs.

Premenstrual dysphoric disorder is a complex condition for which we don't have all the answers. The intense research of the past thirty years has produced some very useful information, which is helping us to understand and recognize PMS and its severe subset, PMDD. We can more easily identify this condition, and guide more women toward interventions that can help them. The balance of this book is devoted to that end.

PART 2

Self-Help Interventions

If you suffer from PMDD or PMS, symptom relief is probably your main goal. Improvement often requires a combination of treatment approaches including lifestyle modifications and, for many, drug therapy. We urge you to consult a knowledgeable and caring health advisor with whom you can communicate openly and easily. In such a relationship, you can formulate a plan that focuses on the symptoms that are the most distressing to you.

Our goal in the next few chapters is to give you some weapons to help you combat and prevent PMDD. Though modifying your lifestyle may not be easy, it is often the most effective intervention. The next chapter will explain the general value of healthful nutrition and nutritional supplements, plus some nutritional specifics for PMDD control. Succeeding chapters will cover the influence of weight control and exercise, and alternative medical therapies such as herbal remedies, traditional Chinese medicine, Ayurvedic medicine, homeopathy, naturopathy, and craniosacral therapy.

CHAPTER 3

Nutritional Help
for PMDD

Women who are generally well are less troubled by PMDD/PMS than those who are not. This is because wellness is much more than the mere absence of disease. Wellness also means feeling vigorous, alert, robust, and having the sense that you are in control of your body and your life. Thus, wellness is an important goal for women with PMDD. To achieve and maintain wellness, you must become proactive. Maintaining wellness means becoming focused not only on the symptoms of a condition that distresses you but also on the larger factors that influence your overall health, including adequate nutrition, a balanced diet, weight control, and exercise. These are the topics of this chapter and the next. Stress management, covered in chapter 7, is also important. Our goal is to show you how you can help control your PMDD by taking better care of yourself.

Nutrition

It is well known that diet can affect your health. With PMDD, certain foods can actually decrease your symptoms whereas others can exacerbate them.

First, let's consider each of the food types, called *macronutrients*. Protein, carbohydrates, and fat are the three principal categories of food. Water can be considered a fourth ingredient. Each of these food types contains varying amounts of vitamins and minerals, and each serves an important role in a balanced diet. Nutritionists and food scientists have studied their various effects on the body, and as a result, can recommend the most healthful diet. After we consider the nutritional value of proteins, carbohydrates, fats, minerals, and vitamins, we'll put them together in a nutritional plan.

Protein

Your body can make protein by assembling amino acids into chains. There are twenty-two known amino acids, and your body can make all but nine of them. These nine are known as *essential amino acids*, and they must be supplied by the food you eat. A complete protein is one that supplies all nine essential amino acids. Meat and dairy products are complete proteins; fruits and vegetables are not.

Most nutritionists agree that only 25 percent of your diet should be made up of protein. They recommend that you eat 0.42 grams of protein per pound of *ideal body weight* each day. (You can calculate your own ideal weight using the body mass index discussed in chapter 4.) That comes to 55 grams if your ideal weight is 130 pounds, but most Americans consume much more than that (Ojeda 1995). There are some risks in consuming too much protein. If your intake is more than 50 percent above your daily needs, you may secrete calcium in your urine. You lose this calcium from your bones, which, over time, poses a risk for osteoporosis.

Another problem is that the typical American diet derives most of its protein from meat and dairy products, which are high in fat. High fat intake increases your risk for cardiovascular disease, obesity, and certain cancers. So not enough protein is bad, too much is also bad. You should aim for just right. Look over table 3.1 for a list of commonly consumed protein foods to get a rough estimate of whether you meet the recommended intake. If you are a vigorously active woman (you do daily aerobics or are a proficient athlete), calculate your daily requirement using 0.5 to 1.0 grams per pound instead of 0.42.

Carbohydrates

Carbohydrates influence PMDD. They consist of sugars, starches, and fiber. They are your primary energy source, with fat and protein available as backup sources. Carbohydrates also play a role in determining the severity of PMDD symptoms. Carbohydrates circulate in your blood as a sugar called glucose, and this is your body's first choice when it comes to energy needs. Blood glucose can get used up quickly, though, so your liver converts some of it into a substance called *glycogen* and stores it for resupplying your blood glucose as needed. When your carbohydrate intake is excessively high, and there is far more glucose in your blood than can be burned as energy, it is converted to fat by insulin and stored in your body's fat cells.

Table 3.1. Daily Protein Needs for Women

Formula using ideal weight in pounds: _____ lbs x 0.42 = _____ grams per day

Food Source	Serving	Protein in Grams
Chicken	4 oz	36
Beef	4 oz	32
Fish	4 oz	28
Wheat cereal with milk	1 cup	28
Beans with rice	1 cup	17
Eggs	2	14
Cottage cheese	½ cup	14
Milk	1 cup	9
Cheddar cheese	1 oz	7
Beans	½ cup	7
Pasta	1 cup	5
Potato	1 medium	5
Whole wheat bread	1 slice	3

Adapted from: Ojeda 1995.

Your body can make carbohydrates from components of protein and fat, so there aren't any essential carbohydrates. The three types of carbohydrates—simple sugars and refined carbohydrates, complex carbohydrates, and fiber—have differing effects on your body and your health.

Simple Sugar and Refined Carbohydrate— Bad for PMDD

A high simple sugar intake increases the prevalence and severity of PMDD/PMS (Rossignol and Bonnlander 1991). Simple sugars appear naturally in honey and fruit juice, but also in white sugar, sweets, ice cream, chocolate, and most regular soft drinks. They are absorbed directly into your bloodstream without any significant digestive alteration, which is why you get such a quick energy surge from them. Refined carbohydrate foods are those made from white flour, refined sugar, and white rice. They are low in vitamins and minerals, which is bad enough, but the biggest problem with these foods is that they don't contain fiber.

Sugar is a great source of instant energy; but it doesn't last long. When you load up on sugar, your blood glucose rises rapidly. This causes your pancreas to pour out insulin to get your blood glucose under control.

Insulin production often overshoots the mark in reducing your blood sugar, and you end up with too little glucose. Now you feel tired and weak again, so you start the cycle over with another portion of the sugar source.

Complex Carbohydrates and Fiber—PMDD Fighters

Complex carbohydrates contribute significantly to PMDD control. They are chiefly starches found in corn, potatoes, pasta, rice, grains, and beans (lima, navy, kidney), but also in fruits and vegetables. When you eat them in an unrefined state, they provide abundant vitamins, minerals and, especially, fiber. Most nutritionists recommend that complex carbohydrates should constitute 40 to 55 percent of everyone's daily caloric intake (Bland 1999; Daoust and Daoust 1996), but in the typical American diet, it is far lower.

Dietary fiber is the indigestible part of these foods. It is found in the plant cell walls, and it is not absorbed into your bloodstream. Fiber comes in two forms, each of which carries out important functions.

- **Water-soluble fiber** is found in whole grains, barley, oat-bran cereals, and beans, plus many fruits and vegetables. Soluble fiber aids in lowering cholesterol, triglycerides, and harmful low-density lipoproteins (LDL). We will discuss cholesterol in a minute.

- **Insoluble fiber** is predominantly found in whole-wheat products, corn and rice bran, wheat bran, plus the skins and pulp of vegetables and fruits. This is the fiber that softens stools and prevents constipation.

Nutritionists recommend twenty-five to thirty grams of fiber each day, which is in stark contrast to the average fiber-depleted American diet of ten to fifteen grams. There are numerous benefits to an adequate fiber intake.

- **Mood control:** Complex carbohydrates and their fiber assist in controlling the negative moods associated with PMDD and PMS. The reason is that they raise the brain level of an amino acid called *tryptophan*, which is converted to the neurotransmitter *serotonin*. You know from chapter 2 that low serotonin levels are a major contributor to PMDD. Inadequate serotonin also influences sleep patterns, pain perception, and hormone secretion and is associated with depression. So, start your PMDD day with a large bowl of a high carbohydrate cereal, even if you hate the cereal, hate the bowl, hate the spoon, and hate the skim milk you pour over it. Chances are good you'll feel better within an hour or so.

- **Decreased risk of coronary heart disease:** An analysis of the Harvard Nurses' Health Study found that whole grains in breakfast cereal, brown rice, oatmeal, and bran significantly reduce the risk of heart disease. Five or more cereal breakfasts per week are necessary. The fiber in fruits and vegetables was not protective (Harvard Heart Letter 2000).

- **Decreased risk of diabetes:** Fiber takes longer to be broken down than other food components, so it slows the absorption of glucose into your bloodstream. This aids in blood sugar control, and decreases the likelihood of glucose being stored as fat. It also decreases your risk of developing diabetes and helps blood sugar regulation in those who are already diabetic.

- **Decreased cancer risks:** A high-fiber diet has been associated with decreased incidence of colon cancer, although a recent study has cast doubt on this benefit. It may lower the incidence of other cancers as well.

- **Weight control:** High-fiber foods are lower in calories and fat than low-fiber foods. In addition, digestion of fiber is slow, which contributes to your feeling fuller longer.

- **Control of intestinal problems:** Fiber prevents constipation because it absorbs water, creating a softer stool. (Many commercial stool softeners are powdered fiber.)

When you increase your fiber intake, do it gradually. A sudden jump can result in gas and bloating. Drink plenty of water (six to eight cups a day) with your increased fiber diet because there will be more bulk in your intestine and, without water accompanying it, you can become constipated. One more precaution is to be aware that fiber can prevent or decrease the absorption of calcium and iron. If you are using these supplements, do not take them at the same time as a high-fiber meal. Table 3.2 lists the fiber content of common foods. When you select breads and cereals, use whole-grain products. Refining these grains removes 60 to 90 percent of the vitamins, minerals, and fiber (Willet 1994).

Fat

Fat is a necessary ingredient in your diet. Fat is a very concentrated source of energy since it contains nine calories per gram, as compared to four calories per gram in both proteins and carbohydrates. Fat storage represents a valuable warehouse for energy and water to which your body can turn when supplies are otherwise low. Fat cushions vital organs from injury and insulates your body from cold. Dietary fat aids in the absorption of the fat-soluble vitamins A, D, E, and K. Fat makes your food taste

Table 3.2. Fiber Content of Various Foods

Type of Food

	Serving	Fiber in Grams
Cereals		
All Bran with extra fiber	½ cup	14.0
All Bran	½ cup	12.9
100% Bran	½ cup	10.0
Raisin Bran	¾ cup	5.3
40% Bran Flakes	½ cup	4.3
Oat bran, cooked	¾ cup	4.0
Oat bran cereal, cold	¾ cup	2.9
Corn flakes	¾ cup	2.1
Special K	¾ cup	1.2
Cream of Wheat	¾ cup	0.5
Rice Krispies	¾ cup	0
Breads		
Pita bread, whole wheat	1.5-inch pocket	4.4
Pumpernickel	1 slice	2.7
Whole wheat	1 slice	1.5
Bagel, plain	1	1.4
White bread, French, Italian	1 slice	0.6
Croissant	1	0
Legumes (Beans and Peas)		
Black-eyed peas, cooked	¾ cup	12.3
Kidney or pinto beans, cooked	¾ cup	14.0
Kidney beans, canned	¾ cup	4.7
Lima beans, cooked	½ cup	3.5
Lentils, cooked	½ cup	5.2
Split peas, cooked	½ cup	3.1
Peas, canned	½ cup	2.8
Fruits		
Apple, large, with skin	1	4.7
Apricots, dried	10	3.6
Orange	1 medium	3.0
Pear, with skin	1 small	2.9
Peach, with skin	1 medium	2.0

Fruits, cont.

Prune, dried	3 medium	1.7
Raspberries, fresh	½ cup	1.7
Grapefruit, medium	½	1.4
Pineapple, canned	½ cup	1.2
Banana, medium	1	0.7
Raisins	2 tbsp	0.4
Grapes, green, fresh	½ cup	0.4
Vegetables		
Peas, green, cooked	½ cup	4.3
Potato, baked, with skin	1 medium	4.2
Brussels sprouts, cooked	½ cup	3.8
Corn, whole, cooked	½ cup	3.0
Carrots, raw	1 medium	2.3
Broccoli, cooked	½ cup	1.5
Spinach, raw	1 cup	1.4
Tomato, cooked	½ cup	1.0
Lettuce, iceberg	1 cup	0.6

Adapted from: Ojeda 1995; Cutler 1992

good. And because it digests more slowly than other foods, fat also gives you that pleasant feeling of fullness after a meal. That is the good news about fat. The bad news is that we eat too much of it.

On average, Americans consume about 34 percent of their daily calories from dietary fat (McDowell et al. 1994). Some have estimated the level to be as high as 40 percent. The number should actually be about 25 to 30 percent, to meet your body's needs and to remain healthy. A high-fat diet contributes to obesity, and raises your risk of cardiovascular disease, high blood pressure, diabetes, and certain cancers.

Fat Types

There are several types of dietary fat. Too much of any of them is not good for you, but some are worse than others. All fats are composed of fatty acids, which are chemicals that are put together in a variety of ways to make each type. Saturated fats and hydrogenated fats are the main troublemakers. Monounsaturated and polyunsaturated fats are less harmful.

Triglycerides are another form of fat that your liver makes from the food you eat. We discuss each of them below.

Saturated fat. Dietary enemy number one. Your primary source is animal foods and dairy products. Most saturated fats are solid at room temperature: butter, cheese, lard, meat fat, and chocolate. Some are liquid: coconut oil, palm oil, and cream. Cholesterol has gotten a bad name because foods high in saturated fat are also laden with cholesterol. A diet high in cholesterol does not necessarily raise the blood cholesterol if saturated fat intake is low. That means eating one to two eggs per day is okay as long as your consumption of saturated fat and trans fatty acids (to be discussed) is low (Hu 1999). On the other hand, a high saturated-fat diet raises "bad" LDL (low-density lipoproteins) cholesterol and significantly increases the risk of heart and vascular disease.

Your daily calorie intake from fat should be less than 10 percent from saturated fat. If your cholesterol is abnormally high, saturated fat should constitute less than 7 percent of your daily calories (Johns Hopkins Health Letter 2001).

Hydrogenated fat (trans fatty acids). Hydrogenation is a chemical process that converts naturally occurring oils like coconut and peanut oil to saturated fat. Margarine and shortenings use hydrogenated fat. Hydrogenated oils are used in many processed products, such as corn chips, baked goods, potato chips, and deep-fried foods. Trans fatty acids are just as bad as saturated fat in raising your bad LDL, but even worse, they also lower your good HDL (high-density lipoproteins), which saturated fat does not do. One study showed a 66 percent higher risk of heart disease in women who used margarine four or more times daily compared to women who used it almost not at all (Willet, Stampfer, and Manson 1993).

Polyunsaturated fats. These are vegetable derivatives of cottonseed, corn, safflower, sunflower, soybeans, and wheat germ. They are generally liquid at room temperature. Polyunsaturated fats lower blood levels of cholesterol and bad LDL, but they also lower good HDL so it's a mixed blessing. Monounsaturated oils are considered safer.

Monounsaturated fats. Monounsaturated fats are vegetable products contained in olive oil, peanut oil, and canola oil, which have no undesirable effects on cholesterol. As a matter of fact, they make LDL cholesterol more resistant to oxidation, which reduces the tendency for cholesterol to be deposited on artery walls. This is a definite plus. If you are choosing between olive oil and butter, go for the olive oil. But don't make olive oil a net addition to your fat intake. If you are going to emphasize olive oil in your diet, cut back on something else, like meats and poultry. Too much fat is too much fat, no matter what form it takes.

Triglycerides. Most foods that contain fat have triglycerides. You store it in fat cells as an energy reservoir. The significance of this fat to you as a woman is that high levels in your blood pose much more of a risk for coronary heart disease than the same levels in men (Lapidus 1986).

Fish oils. Omega-3 fatty acids, found in fish oils, are a polyunsaturated fat found in a large variety of fish. Sardines are very high in omega-3 fatty acids, but other excellent sources with lesser amounts are sockeye salmon, Atlantic mackerel, albacore tuna, herring, and halibut (Bellerson 1993). Studies of Greenland Eskimos showed their traditionally high-fish diets resulted in less than half the heart attack rate of that experienced in the United States even though the cholesterol levels were about the same in both populations (Kromhaut, Bosschieter, and Coulander 1985). This benefit was traced to the omega-3 fatty acids in fish oil. These fatty acids lower triglyceride levels quite effectively. They also have a beneficial influence on clotting factors, which is thought to be part of the reason for the lowered heart attack rate in the study.

More recently, a Danish study found that daily fish oil and vitamin B_{12} supplements reduced premenstrual complaints such as cramps, nausea, fatigue, and headaches. The benefit lasted up to three months after discontinuing the fish oil and B_{12}. Does this mean you should eat a lot of fish? The researchers concluded that eating as little as one or two servings of fish a week gave as much protection as a high-fish diet (Albert et al. 1998). They also found that concentrated fish oil use will lower your triglycerides, but actually may raise your undesirable LDL. The current recommendation is to avoid fish oil capsules, and to rely on fish consumption for the known benefits.

What about Cholesterol?

Cholesterol isn't really a fat. It is a *lipid*, a waxy substance found in animal foods and dairy products. As you know, cholesterol plays a major role in hardening of the arteries (atherosclerosis), resulting in cardiovascular disease. Cholesterol itself, however, is not harmful; indeed it is vital to your existence. Cholesterol helps build cell membranes (all three trillion of them). Cholesterol is also the basic building block for hormones. Your body uses it to make vitamin D. Cholesterol forms a protective sheath around nerves, which facilitates transmission of impulses, and it serves many, many other important biologic functions. Your body can manufacture all the cholesterol it needs, but the problem is that you add to the supply from the foods you eat. If your cholesterol intake is too high, the level of cholesterol in your blood rises. Then you start depositing the excess amounts of this waxy substance on the walls of arteries, which leads to hardening of your arteries, high blood pressure, and coronary heart disease.

Cholesterol is carried to your body's cells in your bloodstream. The carrier substances, or lipoproteins, are manufactured in your liver by combining fat and protein, to which cholesterol is attached. There are several types of lipoproteins, but two are especially important.

- *High-density lipoproteins* (HDL): This is "good cholesterol," so-called because HDL carries cholesterol away from the artery walls to the liver for harmless elimination from your body

- *Low-density lipoproteins* (LDL): This is "bad cholesterol" which is deposited on artery walls if blood levels of it are too high

Table 3.3 lists the amount of cholesterol in many common foods.

Influence of Vitamins and Minerals on PMDD

Thousands of dietary supplements are on the market. Many contain vitamins and minerals to supplement similar nutrients you get in food you eat. Many others, such as herbs, other botanicals, enzymes, and animal extracts, contain substances that may have a high potency and be potentially dangerous if used incorrectly. The FDA puts less time into reviewing supplements than it does for drugs and other products it regulates, so it pays to be cautious about using supplements that claim to treat, prevent, or cure a disease. The Dietary Supplement Health and Education Act, enacted by Congress in 1994, specifically prohibits such claims.

Research does indicate, however, that certain vitamins and minerals may help diminish or eliminate premenstrual symptoms. We have summarized them in the list that follows.

Vitamin B_6 (pyridoxine). This vitamin is a co-factor in the synthesis of serotonin and prostaglandins. As you know, adequate serotonin levels are necessary for mood control. Prostaglandins are chemicals manufactured throughout the body that exert a hormone-like effect and influence involuntary muscle contraction (including uterine menstrual cramps). B_6 has been found to be helpful for premenstrual symptoms in doses of 50 to 100 milligrams per day, but it is necessary to take it all month, not just premenstrually. Some food supplement advocates suggest 100 to 400 milligrams per day, but you should exercise caution because larger doses can result in irreversible nerve damage. Such damage has been reported in as little as 200 milligrams per day (Parker 1994). In a composite report of several controlled trials, women who used B_6 reported relief from premenstrual symptoms twice as often as those using the placebo (Wyatt et al. 1999).

Table 3.3   Calories, Fat, and Cholesterol in Foods

Food	Serving	Calories	Fat (grams)	Cholesterol (mgs)
Candy				
Milk chocolate bar	1 oz	150	9.2	5
Cheese				
Cheddar	1 oz	112	9.1	30
Cottage, 2% fat	½ cup	100	2.2	9
Monterey jack	1 oz	105	8.5	30
Swiss, pasteurized	1 oz	95	7.1	26
Cheese Whiz spread	1 oz	80	6.0	15
Condiments				
Mayonnaise	1 tbsp	100	11.0	5
Diet mayonnaise	1 tbsp	45	5.0	5
Miracle Whip	1 tbsp	70	7.0	5
Dairy Products				
Whole milk	1 cup	150	8.1	34
Low-fat milk	1 cup	122	4.7	20
Skim milk	1 cup	89	0.4	5
Yogurt, nonfat	1 cup	127	0.4	4
Yogurt, whole milk	1 cup	141	7.7	30
Egg, whole	1 med	78	5.5	250
Egg yolk	1 med	59	5.2	250
Egg Beaters	¼ cup	25	0	0
Fats & Oils				
Butter	1 tbsp	108	12.2	36
Margarine	1 tbsp	108	12.0	0
Vegetable oil	1 tbsp	120	13.5	0
Butter Buds	1 oz	12	0	0
Molly McButter	1 tsp	5	0	0
Seafood				
Crab, king	3½ oz	93	1.9	60
Fish sticks, frozen	3½ oz	176	8.9	70
Lobster	3½ oz	91	1.9	100
Mackerel	3½ oz	191	12.2	95
Oysters	3½ oz	66	1.8	50
Salmon	3½ oz	182	7.4	47

Continued on the following page

| | | | Table 3.3. cont. | |
Food	Serving	Calories	Fat (grams)	Cholesterol (mgs)
Seafood (cont.)				
Sardines, canned in oil	3½ oz	311	24.4	120
Shrimp	3½ oz	91	0.8	100
Tuna, canned in oil	3½ oz	197	8.2	63
Tuna, canned in water	3½ oz	127	0.8	63
Breads				
English muffin	1	133	1.0	0
Pita, pocket	1	145	1.0	0
White	1 slice	68	0.8	0
Whole wheat	1 slice	61	0.8	0
Meats				
Beef, trimmed, cooked	3 oz	192	9.4	73
Ground beef, 27% fat	3 oz	251	16.9	86
Ground beef, 10% fat	3 oz	213	11.9	86
Lamb chop	3 oz	188	8.9	82
Pork chop	3 oz	219	12.7	80
Spareribs	3 oz	338	25.8	103
Bacon	1 slice	40	3.0	5
Ham, 3% fat	3 oz	120	6.0	45
Chicken, light, no skin	3 oz	153	4.2	66
Chicken, with skin	3 oz	210	12.6	75
Turkey, light, no skin	3 oz	153	4.2	66
Turkey, with skin	3 oz	210	12.6	75
Veal, lean only	3 oz	120	2.7	84
Beef liver	3½ oz	140	4.7	300
Beef brain	3½ oz	106	7.3	2100
Bologna	1 oz	88	8.1	15+
Canadian bacon	1 oz	45	2.0	13
Liverwurst	1 oz	139	9.1	35
Salami	1 oz	112	9.8	22
Hot dog	1.6 oz	142	13.5	23
Salad Dressing				
Blue Cheese	1 tbsp	71	7.3	4–10
Russian	1 tbsp	74	7.6	7–10
French	1 tbsp	66	6.2	0
Italian	1 tbsp	83	9.0	0

vitamin E. Several small studies have shown that vitamin E supplements at 600 to 800 international units (IU) per day are effective for premenstrual breast pain and tenderness in about 85 percent of women (Severino and Moline 1995). The mechanism through which vitamin E improves symptoms is not known, but it may involve regulation of prostaglandin synthesis or neurotransmitters. Toxic levels of vitamin E are 3,000 IU per day, so the safety margin is adequate.

Calcium. Calcium is your body's most important mineral. It is vital to bone integrity, but also necessary for proper nerve transmission of impulses, proper muscle functioning (including heart muscle), the blood clotting mechanism, and many other bodily needs. A large multicenter study found that 1,200 milligrams of calcium per day (through food and supplements, if needed) was effective for nearly 48 percent of women in reducing premenstrual depression, fatigue, food cravings, water retention, pain, and insomnia (Thys-Jacobs et al. 1998). The proposed explanation for calcium's benefit in PMDD is that it restored a calcium deficit (most women get less than half the daily recommendation of calcium), reduced muscle spasms, and suppressed overactive parathyroid hormone activity. (If calcium is too low in your blood, the parathyroid tries to supply it by removing calcium from your bones). Toxic levels of calcium are not reached until 2,500 milligrams per day (Institute of Medicine 1997). Calcium absorption decreases when you have too much protein, oxalic acid foods (dark-green leafy veggies), or alcohol in your diet. Dietary fiber binds calcium and prevents absorption, so don't take your calcium supplement with a high fiber meal.

Magnesium. Magnesium may reduce premenstrual symptoms through its effect on the regulation of serotonin and other neurotransmitters (Bendich 2000). One small study found that 1,080 milligrams of magnesium daily reduced fluid retention, which causes weight gain, breast tenderness, ankle swelling, and abdominal bloating (Fachinetti et al. 1991). This is twice the recommended daily dose. In addition to causing loose bowel movements, this dosage can interfere with calcium absorption and pose a risk for osteoporosis in later years. Therefore, you should use this level of magnesium supplementation only premenstrually. Cut the dose back as soon as your menstrual period starts. A more recent controlled study using 200 milligrams of magnesium daily reported a significant reduction in premenstrual fluid retention (Walker, DeSouza, and Vickers 1998). It takes two to three cycles for the effects of magnesium to be established.

Be cautious in using diuretics (water pills) because they deplete magnesium.

Potassium. Potassium may help alleviate premenstrual symptoms. A preliminary uncontrolled study found that women with PMDD had complete resolution of their symptoms in four cycles (Takacs 1998). In the year-long trial, 400 milligrams of potassium gluconate plus 200 milligrams of potassium chloride were used daily in the first two cycles. Then all participants switched to 600 milligrams of potassium gluconate for the balance of the study. There was a gradual improvement in bloating, fatigue, irritability, and other symptoms over a four-month period, after which all women became symptom-free. This is quite remarkable, of course, so the world awaits the results of controlled trials to confirm these findings.

Manganese. A small study found that manganese levels vary throughout the menstrual cycle. Women with low dietary manganese intake reported increased mood and pain symptoms premenstrually, which were relieved with supplements of six milligrams of manganese per day (Penland and Johnson 1993). The usual recommended daily dose is 1.8 milligrams (Daugherty 1998). No other studies have been published on this topic, so the benefit of this supplement remains uncertain.

L-tryptophan. L-tryptophan is an amino acid found in most common proteins, especially dairy products, meat, soy protein, pumpkin, sesame seeds, and lentils. L-tryptophan precursors are also found in complex carbohydrates. L-tryptophan has been found to significantly reduce premenstrual irritability, tension, mood swings, fluid retention, breast tenderness, and headache. This is because your body converts it to serotonin (Steinberg 1999). Unfortunately, L-tryptophan was removed from the market in 1991 when several deaths were traced to a contaminant in a batch made in Japan. It was the contaminant in the batch, not the L-tryptophan, that caused the problem, but the FDA banned it as an unapproved experimental drug.

A modified form of tryptophan called 5-hydroxytryptophan (5-HTP) is now available as an over-the-counter supplement; 5-HTP is a metabolic by-product of L-tryptophan. While L-tryptophan was made with a fermentation process, 5-HTP is derived from the seed pods of *Griffonia simplicifolia*, a West African plant. Like L-tryptophan, 5-HTP is also converted to serotonin in your body, and has similar beneficial effects on PMDD. The dosage range is 50 to 300 milligrams daily during the premenstrual days of your cycle. (Two problems with 5-HTP are that it may cause drowsiness and can seriously increase the effects of drugs prescribed for mood disorders, such as SSRIs, or drugs to suppress appetite.)

Miscellaneous Vitamin and Mineral Supplements

Several over-the-counter vitamin and mineral supplements are available to treat premenstrual symptoms. Most of them contain vitamin B_6 and recommend multiple tablets throughout the day. Be cautious that you aren't getting more than 100 milligrams of B_6 daily. (Check the dosage on the multivitamin container.) Serious neurological disorders have been reported on as little as 200 milligrams per day.

How Do You Put All This Together?

In order for your brain chemicals to be at optimum levels to lessen PMDD, it is essential for you to maintain a balanced diet. This means that your total daily calorie intake should be composed of about 40 to 55 percent complex carbohydrates, 25 percent protein, and 25 to 30 percent fat.

Serotonin precursors in the form of L-tryptophan are found in complex carbohydrates; so the "carbo-cravings" so common in PMDD/PMS may indicate a natural need to increase serotonin levels. Past recommendations for PMS sufferers were to increase proteins and limit carbohydrates, but it appears to have been the wrong advice. The evidence now is that meals high in complex carbohydrates and low in protein reduce mood symptoms, including anger, tension, depression, fatigue, confusion, and alertness.

We can also make some additional suggestions for maximum PMDD benefit.

- **Avoid a large salt intake:** Most women who experience PMDD/PMS increase their salt and simple carbohydrate (sweets) intake premenstrually and thereby unwittingly increase their premenstrual fluid retention symptoms. Foods high in salt include cured meats, canned foods, frozen dinners, cheese, mustard, soy sauce, packaged sauces, pickled foods, chips, and salted nuts.

- **Limit sugar:** It is common to crave sweets as your menstrual period approaches, but you should try not to give in to it. A high intake of sweets causes salt retention in your body. The increased salt in turn causes fluid retention and increases premenstrual bloating and weight gain. So, when you feel the urge to eat sweets, eat some complex carbohydrates instead. You need to limit sweets and eat more grains, vegetables, pastas, and fruits. These are all complex carbohydrates that will help relieve your symptoms.

- **Increase your fluid intake:** Fluid retention and bloating are common premenstrual complaints. Many women gain more than five pounds each month. You might think that if you severely restricted your salt intake, water retention would be reduced. This sounds like it would work, but it doesn't. The solution to fluid retention and bloating, surprisingly enough, is to increase your water intake. Hard to believe it works, but it does. Increased water pulls salt from your tissues, and it is eliminated in the urine. The more water you drink, the more salt-laden fluid you flush out (Huston and Lanka 2001).

- **Reduce or eliminate caffeine:** Large amounts of caffeine in coffee, colas, and chocolate make the symptoms of PMDD/PMS worse. Caffeine increases anxiety, tension, depression, and irritability, and contributes to insomnia (Caan, Duncan, and Hiatt 1993).

- **Eliminate or cut down on alcohol:** In its various forms, alcohol may seem like a reasonable choice during PMDD because it tends to relax you. But keep in mind that alcohol is basically a brain depressant, and heavy use can aggravate your down moods. Alcohol also interferes with calcium absorption, which you now know is necessary at about 1,200 milligrams per day to help control PMDD.

- **Stop cigarette smoking:** Nicotine increases anxiety and tension, both of which aggravate PMDD.

- **Avoid strict diets that impose severe menu limitations:** Strict diets are stressful, which adds to PMDD symptoms. You should eat three balanced meals a day, even if you are dieting. Just eat three smaller meals, and some healthy snacks such as raw veggies.

- **Vitamins and minerals:** A daily multivitamin supplement can be helpful in contributing to your overall wellness. If you have PMDD, though, take an additional daily supplement of vitamin B_6 so the total is 50 to 100 milligrams. If you decide to use vitamin E, you will probably need a supplement to reach the recommended 600 to 800 IU level. Be sure that your calcium intake through diet and supplements totals 1,200 milligrams daily throughout the month. Vitamin D is needed for optimum calcium absorption, but there will be a sufficient amount in your multivitamin capsule. In the seven to ten days before your menstrual period is due, supplement your daily diet with 1,080 milligrams of magnesium, but don't forget to cut that dose in half as soon as your menstrual flow begins so that you don't impair calcium absorption.

- **Manganese:** You will have to judge for yourself. The usefulness of manganese has not been clearly demonstrated.

- **5-HTP:** 5-hydroxytryptophan has been shown to be helpful, but be sure your doctor knows you are using this supplement if he or she is prescribing an SSRI (selective serotonin reuptake inhibitor).

Are you getting the impression that no single intervention fixes PMDD? If so, you've got it just about right. But a good diet with appropriate nutritional supplements contributes to your controlling PMDD. This chapter has been about the role that good nutrition plays in your achieving wellness, which in itself diminishes PMDD suffering. In the next chapter we will cover two more elements of self-help intervention: exercise and weight control.

CHAPTER 4

Weight Management and Exercise

In your quest for wellness, weight control and exercise play crucial roles. Both are also important to relieving PMDD. Destructive behaviors such as overeating and a sedentary lifestyle contribute to many illnesses, such as high blood pressure, heart disease, diabetes, stroke, and even cancer. It's also known that these behaviors add to the severity of premenstrual symptoms. Changing long-ingrained habits is not easy, but the physical and psychological benefits can be powerful. Ridding yourself of a destructive lifestyle habit usually translates to a huge boost in self-esteem.

Weight Management

Sixty-one percent of American adults and twenty-five percent of our children are overweight (Women's HealthSource 1999; Centers for Disease Control and Prevention 2000). The percentage of overweight adults, both women and men, is increasing by nearly 1 percent per year. We eat too much.

If you think you have a weight problem, your bathroom scale or a standard weight chart can give you your first clues. The problem is that they only tell you your weight. They fail to distinguish between overweight and overfat. There's a difference. Too much body fat is the real culprit when it comes to obesity-related health risks, such as increased premenstrual symptoms, high blood pressure, heart disease, diabetes, and certain cancers, like colorectal cancer.

Determining your percentage of body fat is the most accurate way to assess your physical shape. This can be done in a variety of ways. One way is to take girth measurements of waist and hips; your hip measurement should be slightly larger in a ratio of 1 to 0.8., meaning your hips should be at least 20 percent greater than your waist in measurement. Another way is to have your body weighed underwater. Ultrasound, dual-energy X-ray absorptiometry (DEXA), CT scans, infrared interactance, and bioelectric impedance scanning are also being used to make these determinations (Roubenoff, Dallal, and Wilson 1995; Women's Health-Source 1999). These are all rather complicated methods that require third-party help in dealing with the numbers. Calculating your *body mass index* is an easier way.

Body-Mass Index (BMI)

Body-mass index estimates your proportion of body fat. Calculate your BMI using the following formula: (Weight in lbs. x 703) ÷ (height in inches squared). If you weigh 130 pounds and are 5 feet 6 inches tall (66 inches), your calculation would be (130 x 703) ÷ (66 x 66) = 20.9

BMI Interpretation:
Underweight = less than 18.5
Normal weight = 18.5 to 24.9
Overweight = 25 to 29.9
Mildly obese = 30.0 to 34.9
Moderately obese = 35 to 39.9
Extremely obese = over 40.0

BMI is being used as the standard for reference levels of body weight for women and men. The drawback is that it is based on averages and fails to take into account differing builds (frame sizes.) Still, it is a reasonable guide for determining whether you may be carrying too much fat.

What Causes Obesity?

Excessive fat storage is the fundamental cause of obesity, but things are more complex than that. Several factors are involved in fat accumulation:

- **Appetite:** The neurotransmitter norepinephrine stimulates hunger; serotonin suppresses it. As you know, low serotonin levels accompany PMDD, and this accounts for the premenstrual food cravings you may experience. For some, obesity results when these neurotransmitter appetite regulators become short-circuited and the wrong signals are sent. It can happen at any age. The only evidence that it has happened in you is a large appetite that you can't attribute to other causes, such as hyperthyroidism.

- **Genetics:** We have a genetic mechanism that controls how much body fat we accumulate. It operates much like a thermostat, in that there is a "fat setting" in the brain that regulates the amount of body fat you maintain. An "obesity" gene, called the "OB" gene, has been located in humans (Baron 1997). The gene controls production of a protein called *leptin*, which sends messages to your brain on the status of your overall body fat content. Leptin, in turn, controls another brain hormone called *neuropeptide Y* (NPY), a potent appetite stimulator. If the gene is defective or missing, leptin is not produced in adequate amounts, and NPY is free to make you inappropriately hungry by stimulating overproduction of norepinephrine, your hunger hormone. If your brain is insensitive to leptin, the fat setting may be too high, and obesity results. Research is underway to develop products that will increase the brain's sensitivity to leptin.

- **Gender:** Women of normal weight have an average of 22 percent body fat, as compared to 16 percent in men. Men have a larger muscle mass than women, so men burn 10 to 20 percent more calories than women, even at rest. Because your body burns fewer calories than a man's, it accepts fat more readily, meaning you can gain weight more easily, and it may be more difficult to lose it.

- **Metabolism:** Your metabolism plays a definite role. One factor is your muscle status. Muscle tissue is your main calorie burner. The more muscle you have, the more calories you burn. Another metabolic factor is an enzyme in fat cells called *lipoprotein lipase* (LPL). This enzyme removes triglycerides from your bloodstream and tucks them into fat cells for energy storage. LPL increases during dieting—your body is trying to prevent weight loss. This supports the genetic theory that we are all preprogrammed to have a certain amount of body fat.

- **Aging:** As you age, your metabolism slows down. After age thirty, women start losing about 1 percent of their muscle mass each year as a result of lessened physical activity. This amounts to about one pound per year. With each lost pound of muscle, you burn fifty fewer calories per day. If your caloric intake remains unchanged as time passes, you end up consuming more calories than you burn, and the excess becomes stored as fat. By the time you have lost as much as five pounds of muscle mass, your body is storing 250 calories a day. If your daily calorie intake remains the same, you can gain up to twenty pounds in a year.

Hormones and Weight Change

Several hormones influence weight gain and loss.

Thyroid hormone. Thyroid levels are influenced by what you eat. Production of T4, the metabolically active thyroid hormone, decreases during fasting. This is one reason your metabolic rate slows down during a weight-loss diet. Your body is trying to conserve its energy resources and resist losing tissue, whether it be fat or muscle. Some diet programs use thyroid supplements to counteract this normal effect, but this is at the risk of increasing calcium loss, which increases your risk of developing osteoporosis. Overeating increases production of T4, which raises your metabolic rate in an effort to burn some of the excess calories. However, this weak regulatory effort by your thyroid gland does not work well enough to be a major player in weight control.

Insulin. Produced in the pancreas, insulin unlocks cells for storage of glucose from your bloodstream. Blood glucose is stored as a substance called *glycogen* in your liver and muscles, from where it can be readily accessed and reconverted to glucose for energy needs. But while insulin is necessary, it also plays a major role in causing obesity. It has been called the "supervillain" of obesity (Daoust and Daoust 1996). The problem with insulin arises when there is a glucose overload from a high dietary intake of carbohydrates. Since insulin is thirty times more effective in moving glucose into fat than into muscle, carbohydrate excess results in an insulin surge, with fat storage and weight gain. Over time, cells exposed to high insulin levels can become insensitive to it, a condition known as *insulin resistance*. The result is that high levels, called *hyperinsulinemia*, occur in the blood stream. Chronic high insulin levels cause obesity, clogged arteries, high blood pressure, heart attacks, strokes, increased risk of cancer, diabetes, and accelerated aging in all cells. So this hormone is the kingpin of Americans becoming fat simply because of excessive carbohydrates in their diet. Are you confused by our previous emphasis on complex carbohydrates to help your PMDD symptoms? That advice still holds. Just don't consume the carbs with both hands.

Glucagon. This pancreatic hormone is released in response to *protein* consumption. It regulates the release of glycogen in a steady fashion so blood glucose levels remain stable. The big story is that glucagon also releases fat for use as energy, so it can be regarded as your friendly fat-burning hormone. Glucagon has an inverse relationship with insulin, meaning a high insulin level results in low glucagon (Schwarzbein 1999). Can you see where this is leading? Too much carbohydrate and not enough protein result in high insulin levels with accompanying fat storage, as well as too little glucagon and less fat-burning capability. Bingo—weight gain.

Human growth hormone (hGH). This is a pituitary hormone that is released in response to exercise. It is your body's most powerful fat-burning hormone. Since none of us exercise for long periods of time, hGH doesn't exert a great effect on weight control. But high insulin levels suppress hGH. We trust that you are becoming convinced that insulin is indeed the supervillain of overweight.

Hormone Balance

With the understanding that insulin minimizes burning of fat by causing carbohydrates to be converted to fat and stored in fat cells, it is easy to see how your dietary balance, or imbalance, can result in either an ideal body composition or a compromise of your health. A high carbohydrate intake increases production of insulin, which stores some of the carbohydrate in fat cells, and forces glucose, instead of fat, to be used for energy. But a moderate carbohydrate diet combined with more protein allows glucagon to release fat for energy and protects your body from too much insulin. Hormones regulate virtually everything your body does. All of your body's hormones are interconnected and interdependent upon each other to regulate your functioning in a fashion that maintains optimum health.

Weight Reduction

Approximately 40 percent of American women are on a diet at any given time, even if their weight is normal (Horm and Anderson 1993). The problem is that in the long run, diets don't work, and the stress of dieting aggravates PMDD symptoms. The implication of the word "diet" is that it has a beginning and an end. You start a weight-loss diet to shed a specific amount of weight, which you accomplish on a particular diet plan, and then the diet is over. A high percentage of people will regain most of the lost weight within a year, and all of it within three to five years (Institute of Medicine 1995). Many end up weighing more than they originally had. When you resume normal eating habits, your lipoprotein lipase enzyme, discussed earlier in this chapter, is still programmed to take as much of the triglycerides as possible from the food you eat, refilling those fat cells you so recently emptied. This often leads to another round of dieting, and another cycle of loss and regain.

Part of the reason for this up-and-down pattern of weight change is that losing weight does not eliminate fat cells. Your body contains about 30 billion permanent fat cells, which hold about 135,000 calories, and serve a vital energy storage function (Notelovitz and Tonnessen 1993). Your fat cells can sustain your body's energy needs for about six to seven weeks, even without any food. When all 30 billion of them are full, however, and you are still overeating, your body makes even more fat cells and those cells are permanent as well.

Another reason why you regain weight is that a weight-loss diet reduces your muscle mass. Weight loss from a diet is 75 percent fat (which is good), but 25 percent is lean muscle mass (which is bad) (Kayman, Bravold, and Stern 1990). Since muscle is your main calorie burner, you will probably gain weight when you return to your post-diet "normal" eating habits. Your body is less likely to burn the increased calories and much more likely to store them as fat.

For all these reasons, dieting cannot be relied upon to control your weight and it *can* aggravate your PMDD. This does not mean you should not reduce your caloric intake to lose excess pounds. Calorie cutting is a powerful tool in weight loss. The point, though, is that success hinges on your adopting a weight control program that incorporates foods you will keep in your diet for the rest of your life. This is not a "diet" in the usual sense of the word, because it is not temporary. It is a new way of life. A new eating program can be a reliable way to lose weight permanently—and it is especially reliable if combined with exercise.

Weight-Loss Principles

The key to a weight-losing plan is not only to reduce the total amount of calories you consume, but also to maintain the proportions of macronutrient foods in the "balanced diet" range we discussed in chapter 3, namely 40 to 55 percent complex carbohydrates, 25 percent proteins, 25 to 30 percent fats. Calorie counting is a discouraging pain in the neck, so don't bother with it other than to make an initial determination of how many calories your body needs to maintain ideal weight. Table 4.1 shows you how to calculate the amount of calories you need to maintain a stable weight. For a 130-pound moderately active woman, this amounts to about 1,800 calories per day. To reduce your weight, you can rely on smaller serving sizes for a daily reduction of 500–1,000 calories. Such a calorie reduction will result in about a one-pound loss per week. Look over table 4.2 for meaningful serving sizes.

Table 4.1 Daily Caloric Needs for Women	
General Activity Level	**Daily Calorie Intake**
Sedentary	Ideal weight x 11
Moderately active	Ideal weight x 14
Active	Ideal weight x 18
Adapted from: Ojeda 1995	

Table 4.2   Serving Size Equivalents

Food Serving	Equivalent
3 ounces meat or fish	Deck of cards
Cup of vegetables	Size of your fist
Medium apple	Size of a baseball
½ cup cooked pasta	Ice cream scoop
1½ ounces cheese	Pair of dice
1 teaspoon butter, jelly	End of your thumb
1 cup dry cereal	Large handful

Your dietary composition must be such that maximum fat burning takes place. To do this, remember that insulin control is the key to avoiding fat storage and allowing glucagon to release fat for energy use. This means that excessively high carbohydrate intakes must be avoided. It also means you need adequate protein.

Please keep in mind that these proportions will also serve to help control your PMDD symptoms. A major point we wish to make is that attempting to stick with a stringent weight-losing diet may significantly aggravate PMDD. Fad diets and crash diets can create stress, which you certainly wish to avoid if you suffer from PMDD. [**Caution:** Do not attempt a diet on your own with fewer than 1,000 calories; it can be very dangerous. Deaths have been reported as a result of severe caloric restriction (Baron 1997). Such diets have been used for extreme obesity; but they must be under the strict supervision of a physician who understands the potential hazards and can recognize serious problems if they arise.]

Stick with the following general principles:

- **Go slow:** Don't cut calories severely. Losing one pound a week, or two pounds, is about the right pace.

- **Emphasize foods high in nutrients and low in fat and calories:** The best choices are raw vegetables and fruits, plus complex carbohydrates, such as whole-grain breads and cereals, pasta, legumes, and rice. These are the PMDD fighters.

- **Avoid quick-fix crash diet programs:** If they promise weight losses of more than the recommended one to two pounds a week, they are usually counting on your losing water, not fat. It won't last.

- **Eat three meals per day with most of your calories early in the day:** This increases the likelihood that they will be used for energy during the day. Meals just before bedtime result in more fat storage.

- **Take a multivitamin supplement:** This will supply you with the vitamins you may not be getting.

- **Regard your new eating plan and the accompanying exercise program in this chapter as a permanent part of your life.** We can't emphasize this enough.

Should You Use Diet Pills?

A number of diet pills successfully will suppress your appetite, but none of them will keep the weight off. They do not change your internal fat-regulating mechanism, no matter how long you use them. They *can* give you a reasonable jump-start at the beginning of a weight-loss program. If you are significantly overweight (more than 30 percent over your desirable weight), the use of an appetite suppressant drug (ASD) can produce a weight loss in a few weeks that may motivate you to continue on a long-term plan to control your diet. And if you combine such a regimen with exercise, your chances for permanent change will increase. Still, none of the available appetite suppressant drugs has proven to be the magic bullet for treatment of obesity.

Some ASDs enhance serotonin, which dampens appetite, or suppress norepinephrine, the appetite stimulator. Anything that enhances serotonin should be expected to decrease PMDD symptoms. *Sibutrimine*, marketed as Meridia, is a drug that targets both serotonin and norepinephrine. It has been approved for short-term use in people who are more than 30 percent above their desirable weight. Nevertheless, there are no reports regarding a PMDD benefit from the serotonin-enhancing effect of sibutrimine. *Xenical*, marketed as Orlistat, causes a reduction in fat absorption from the intestine by inhibiting the action of lipase, an enzyme necessary for fat absorption (Davidson et al. 1999). Side effects can include gas, cramping, and a bothersome fatty diarrhea. A randomized control trial found those taking xenical lost an average of nine pounds more weight in a year and kept it off longer than a placebo group (Sjostrom 1998). Xenical reduces the absorption of fat soluble vitamins (A, D, E, and K), so a daily multivitamin is recommended.

The food supplement industry is promoting what is called "herbal phen-fen," named after the ASD withdrawn from the market in 1997 because of suspected heart valve damage. Phen-fen was the nickname for a very popular and widely prescribed ASD combination of phentermine and fenfluramine. The food supplement industry quickly took advantage of phen-fen's absence by marketing what was touted as an herbal equivalent. This turned out to be a mixture of St. John's wort, a plant derivative, and ephedra, an ancient Chinese herb known as *ma huang*. St. John's wort elevates serotonin levels and ephedra is a stimulant. St. John's wort is commonly recommended for PMDD, but combining it with ephedra could be a problem. Ephedra has been reported to cause states of severe agitation, seizures, heart rhythm irregularities, heart attacks, strokes, and even deaths (Langreth 1997). The FDA is considering regulation of ephedra as a drug. Metabolife 356 is another herbal product that has garnered extensive publicity as an appetite suppressant. It has eighteen ingredients, with ephedra and caffeine as the main components. Based on its modest benefit, known risks, and lack of long-term safety data, you should not use Metabolife 356 (Barrette 2000).

Pyruvate, a metabolic breakdown product of glucose, is a very highly touted "fat burner" food supplement that appears on many Internet sites. It is said to boost overall weight loss by 37 percent and enhance fat loss by 48 percent. A close look at the early 1990s literature supporting those claims reveals that pyruvate provides, at most, a very small benefit to obese women in a highly controlled bed-rest environment. The small benefits were exaggerated by statistical manipulation (O'Mathuna 1999).

As mentioned earlier, the obesity gene produces a hormone called leptin that attaches to specific brain receptor sites and regulates how much fat your body stores. Obesity results if the receptor sites are insensitive to leptin or if not enough leptin is produced. Leptin (by injection only, unfortunately) is being used in research projects, and several pharmaceutical companies are working on drugs to increase the brain's sensitivity to leptin.

Another approach to obesity control involves *neuropeptide Y* (NPY), a brain chemical that is a potent appetite stimulus. NPY is suppressed by leptin. Researchers are trying to develop a drug that will dampen the desire to eat by preventing NPY from attaching to brain receptor sites.

The bottom line for using currently available drugs to combat obesity is that they are unlikely to result in more than a 5 to 10 percent reduction in body weight. Starting a weight reduction program with such drugs may be initially helpful, but long-term success still depends on permanent changes in your dietary lifestyle.

Try this sometime when you're hungry: drink a glass of water. It's quite common for thirst to be mistaken for hunger.

Exercise—A Must for Weight Management and PMDD Control

If you eat less food, you will lose weight. Eventually, however, your body will start resisting the tissue destruction and start slowing your metabolism. You burn fewer calories, and weight loss slows. A major cause of this metabolic change is the loss of muscle that results from calorie deprivation. Muscle tissue burns more calories than any other. If you lose twenty pounds from dieting alone, a quarter of it will have been muscle mass. You already know that a pound of muscle will burn about fifty calories each day, so losing five pounds of muscle cuts your calorie expenditure by 250 calories every day. The weight loss may be welcome, but your body composition will have been compromised. The answer to this problem is to *exercise* to avoid muscle loss. No weight management program is complete without it.

There are several reasons why exercise plays such a vital role in weight management and PMDD control:

- **Strenuous exercise releases endorphins** in your brain, which generates a feeling of well-being, relieves depression, and helps PMDD symptoms. In a controlled study, PMDD women who jogged twelve miles per week for six months experienced a significant reduction in breast tenderness, fluid retention, depression, and stress (Prior et al. 1997).

- **Physical stamina improves,** and so does mental stamina. Exercise increases your ability to deal with daily stress.

- **Swelling and puffiness in your feet goes down** as muscle contractions in your lower legs force extra fluid out of your tissues and into your bloodstream for elimination by your kidneys. This is why walking, jogging, cycling, and swimming are so helpful in combating premenstrual symptoms.

- **Exercise burns calories** and stimulates production of human growth hormone, a potent fat burner.

- **Exercise keeps your muscles from deteriorating** and preserves your ability to burn calories.

- **Exercise suppresses appetite**. People who exercise regularly eat less.

- **Exercise decreases health risks associated with being overweight.** These include high blood pressure, abnormal lipid profile (high cholesterol, high triglycerides), diabetes, heart disease, and certain cancers.

- **Exercise is the most efficient way to lose weight when combined with fewer calories.** It has long been known that neither exercise nor diet alone is as effective as they are in combination.

- **When you have reached your target weight**, continuing to exercise has been shown to increase the likelihood that you will maintain it.

What Kind of Exercise?

It is important to choose the right type of exercise. Muscle-resistance exercise will keep you from losing vital muscle mass, so it is an important part of the mix (Butts and Price 1994). On the other hand, while free weights and weight machines make for better muscles, they do little to burn fat. You need aerobic activity to accomplish that. Aerobic exercise also benefits PMDD because it releases endorphins.

With weight control and PMDD relief as the goal, you need a type of aerobic exercise that differs from that needed for achieving cardiovascular fitness. Moderate cardiac fitness can be achieved in three to four months with thirty to forty-five minutes of aerobic exercise about four to five times per week (Kayman, Bruvold, and Stern 1990). For PMDD improvement and weight management, exercise needs to be an every day, or almost every day, event.

Aerobic Conditioning

Aerobic exercise increases oxygen consumption. The main objective of aerobic conditioning is to increase the amount of oxygen your body can process in a given amount of time. This is called your *aerobic capacity*. By improving your ability to utilize oxygen in aerobic exercise, you improve the functioning of your respiratory and cardiovascular systems, as well as increase your muscle tone. Calories are burned in the process, too. Aerobic capacity reflects not only the condition of your muscles, but also the condition of your vital organs, so it is the best measure of your body's physical fitness.

Aerobic activity can be anything from walking to running to dancing to climbing stairs. Your choice of activity should be based on your current level of fitness, how it will fit into your lifestyle, and the fitness goals you have set for yourself.

PMDD Exercise

It's true that the most important time for PMDD exercise is during the premenstrual part of your cycle. Nevertheless, your overall feeling of wellness, which in itself diminishes PMDD suffering, will be more consistent if you exercise daily for about thirty minutes throughout the month. Aerobic exercise (walking, jogging, swimming, and biking) is superior to strength training (weight lifting) in reducing premenstrual symptoms (Moline 1993; Pearlstein, Rivera-Tovar, and Frank 1992). Research has shown that frequency, rather than intensity, is more important in relieving your symptoms and increasing your sense of wellness.

Yoga is another form of exercise that can be beneficial. Through gentle stretches, yoga helps to release muscle tension, ease lower back stiffness, regulate breathing, improve circulation, and relieve stress (American Yoga Association 2001).

Weight Control Exercise

The reason for daily exercise to control weight is somewhat different than for PMDD relief. It revolves around your need to burn fat. In the first twenty minutes of aerobic exercise, the energy you expend is provided by glycogen, which is sugar stored in muscle tissue and your liver. It isn't until your glycogen stores are exhausted that your body turns to fat for energy. This means that a longer workout of about forty-five minutes is necessary. For this reason, select a form of exercise that you can sustain for that length of time, such as cycling or walking. You will need to gradually build up to that level if you are unfit or a beginner. It should be low impact, to protect your tendons and joint surfaces; this is especially important if you are overweight. High impact refers to any exercise that involves both feet being off the ground at the same time.

Ideal exercises might be brisk walking around the neighborhood or on a treadmill, and cycling around town or on a stationary unit. Platform step-aerobics and aerobic dance are also excellent as long as they remain low impact. Swimming is good aerobic exercise and great for muscle strengthening, but it is hard to sustain it long enough to get to the fat-burning stage. Watch out for jogging, running, and some forms of aerobic dance; they are high impact and therefore risk injury to your knees, hips, and ankles.

Be sure to alternate aerobic exercise with muscle resistance training to maintain your muscle mass.

General guidelines: The following guidelines for weight control exercise will help if you are overweight:

- **Be sure to warm up first:** If you are overweight, you are probably less flexible, and your muscles and tendons can be more easily injured. For these reasons, start with some slow walking, cycling, or rowing until your heart rate has increased or you have begun to sweat. Then do some stretching exercises. Don't do any exercise that hurts; wait until you have lost some weight and try again. (**Caution:** There is risk of injury in stretching exercises, so be sure to get expert advice before venturing into a program on your own. Learn how to stretch properly, slow and sustained. A stretch should be sustained for about twenty to thirty seconds to be effective.)

- **Underdo it at the beginning:** If your goal is to walk three miles in forty-five minutes, start with something like three blocks in ten minutes, and work up to your goal. Your tolerance for exercise will be considerably less if you are overweight, so you need to develop it. Remember, this is a new lifestyle for you, and there is plenty of time to ease into your new role.

- **Cool down:** Cooling down after exercise is more important if you are overweight because there is a greater tendency for blood to pool in your legs if you stop suddenly. This can make you feel faint or to actually faint. Gradually diminish your level of activity over five to ten minutes, and let your heart rate return to normal before you become inactive.

- **Caution against overheating:** If you are overweight, you will over-heat more readily, especially in the early stages of becoming more active. Avoid hot rooms or, if you are exercising outside, the hot-test hours of the day. Be sure to drink plenty of fluids before and during your workout. Wear loose-fitting, lightweight clothing. Cottons and linens are best because they allow moisture to evapo-rate, which will help cool you off.

In this chapter, we talked about how destructive behaviors such as overeating and a sedentary lifestyle are common human frailties. They are bad choices that can lead to significant health problems and magnify your premenstrual symptoms. If you have chosen them in the past, you can also "unchoose" them.

Next, we will cover some alternative medical therapies that may help you to combat PMDD.

CHAPTER 5

Integrative Medical Therapies

Despite significant advances in the understanding and treatment of PMDD, many women are frustrated by the obstacles they face in appropriate diagnosis and management of their premenstrual symptoms. One survey found that the majority of women sought help from multiple providers for more than five years before a PMDD or PMS diagnosis was made (Kraemer and Kraemer 1998). As a result, many women look beyond their regular physicians to practitioners of alternative disciplines for management of their symptoms.

In this chapter we will cover methods of dealing with PMDD/PMS that are less well studied and less well proven, but which *can* be helpful for many women. Besides botanical (herbal) remedies, we will look into homeopathy, naturopathy, traditional Chinese medicine, Ayurvedic medicine, and craniosacral therapy, all of which may help women who suffer from PMDD. For further resources, see appendix B.

Botanical Remedies for PMDD

Numerous herbs and other botanical products are used for PMDD/PMS. Many are helpful, and many are not. Because of poor study design and failure to test a botanical substance against a placebo, their effectiveness has not been proven in many cases and exaggerated claims abound (Hardy 2000). It is important to recognize that herbs and many other botanical remedies are regarded as food supplements by the FDA, and are not held to a standard of having to prove either safety or effectiveness. Using herbal remedies is serious business, so it is prudent to be cautious. As the use of unfamiliar botanicals spreads, it is increasingly important for health care professionals and the general public to become familiar with the truly useful preparations as well as the ineffective and dangerous ones.

A common public perception is that herbs cannot cause harm because they are "natural." So are many poisons. It is true that herbal preparations are less concentrated than prescription medications because most prescription drugs contain a single active ingredient. The argument is that herbal preparations are buffered by the many other compounds contained in them and are therefore safe. Indeed, a staggering variety of active ingredients may be present in an herb that can have profound effects, both good and bad. Interaction of herbs with other prescription drugs can seriously increase a drug's effect, resulting in overmedication, or block its effect. Some herbs produced in Asia may contain dangerous levels of lead or other heavy metals, making them toxic and extremely dangerous. The California Department of Health found that 32 percent of 260 Asian products tested contained undeclared chemical ingredients or heavy metals (Ko 1998).

A major problem with botanicals is standardization. Many labels say "standardized" and suggested doses are usually specified. The problem is there may be many active ingredients in a single herb, and much of what they contain is guesswork. Since manufacturers of botanicals are not required to prove either safety or effectiveness, there is little incentive to adopt the rules governing standardization of drugs. Nevertheless, you are better off if the label bears the words "standardized" or "German standards." (German experience with botanicals is quite extensive.)

If herbs are recommended by your health advisor, be certain to disclose any drugs you are taking. And let your physician know about herbs you are using. You and your health advisor need to know what you are doing if herbs are to make a valuable contribution. Herbs need to be properly identified (mistakes are common), capable of maintaining their potency (many do not), clearly labeled for proper indications and contraindications, and prescribed, as well as used, in proper doses.

It is not practical to list all the botanicals that various practitioners may recommend. The following represent those most commonly advocated.

Evening Primrose Oil

This herb contains the essential fatty acid g-linolenic acid. The rationale for using evening primrose oil for premenstrual symptoms is the theory that PMDD involves a deficit of g-linolenic acid resulting in impaired incorporation of essential fatty acids into cell membranes (Johnson 1998).

Several trial studies comparing evening primrose oil with a placebo found the oil reduced premenstrual breast tenderness, but there was no benefit for other symptoms (Khoo, Munro, and Battistutta 1990; Kleijnenn 1994; Budeiri, Li Wan Po, and Doman 1996).

Chaste Tree Berry

Chasteberry gets its name from the belief that the plant would inspire chastity. Monks in ancient Mediterranean cultures would eat it to suppress their sexual desire. It has been used in Europe for many years to treat premenstrual syndrome, menstrual abnormalities, estrogen deficiency complaints (hot flashes), and sore breasts (Robbers 1999). The herb was rated as either very good, good, or satisfactory for premenstrual symptoms by 92 percent of women in one study (Hardy 2000). A German study of 440 women assessed mood changes, anger, breast tenderness, headache, and bloating; 52 percent of the chaste tree berry extract users reported improvement in premenstrual symptoms compared to 24 percent in the placebo group (Schellenberg 2001). In a controlled study, chasteberry was shown to be as effective as 200 milligrams of vitamin B_6 in controlling premenstrual symptoms (Lauritzen, Reuter, and Repges 1997). This herb is unsafe in pregnancy and should not be used if you are trying to become pregnant, or are sexually active without using a reliable form of birth control (Blumenthal, Busse, and Goldberg 1998).

St. John's Wort

Hypericin is the primary active ingredient in this herb and is thought to enhance serotonin levels by inhibiting its reuptake by nerve cells. As you already know, adequate serotonin is key to improving PMDD moods. Numerous other central nervous system activities may involve hypericin because it not only reduces premenstrual symptoms but also seems to help with mild depression. Because St. John's wort eases depressive symptoms, it is being studied for possible beneficial effects in PMDD. So far, one small study of nineteen women in England found that symptoms became about half as bothersome if St. John's wort was used.

Be aware that this herb reduces the effect of blood thinners such as aspirin and warfarin (Coumadin). Interaction with oral contraceptives may cause breakthrough bleeding or reduce their effectiveness in preventing pregnancy (Wellness Letter 2000a). In addition, St. John's wort has an adverse effect on the tumor suppressor gene BRCA1, which can increase the risk of breast and ovarian cancer in women who inherit a mutated form of this gene. This herb can cause photosensitivity; it can make you more sensitive to bright light and make you more susceptible to sunburn.

Valerian Root

Surveys place valerian root as the tenth most popular herb in the United States (Brevcort 1998). It is a mild and effective sedative and sleep aid that is generally recognized as safe. Different valerian species are not equivalent, so the European variant, *Valeriana officinalis L*, is the type most often used (Hardy 1999). Valerian root should not be used with barbiturates or other sedatives, since the combination can cause excessive sedation. Extended use has been associated with dependency and withdrawal symptoms similar to the benzodiazepine tranquilizers (Garges 1998).

Black Cohosh

This botanical, also known as squaw root, is an herb Native Americans have traditionally used for menstrual cramps. It is thought to contain substances that relieve pain and act as sedatives. There is sufficient phytoestrogenic (estrogen-like plant chemical) activity to improve hot flashes and diminish vaginal atrophy in women who have estrogen insufficiency. Because no studies exist on the risk for endometrial cancer with this herb, it is recommended that it be used no longer than three to six months (Tyler 1997). Black cohosh is approved in Germany for treating premenstrual symptoms, but few doctors are recommending it for this purpose since long-term studies of its effectiveness have not be completed (Blumenthal, Busse, and Goldberg 1998).

Ginseng

Ginseng is a widely advertised herb with estrogenic properties. It is sometimes combined with dong quai (see the following discussion) and used for premenstrual disorders, depression, insomnia, nervousness, depressed sexual desire, hot flashes, chronic fatigue, and as a tonic for the elderly. One Web site advertises ginseng to treat a large variety of ailments, from the common cold to Alzheimer's disease to HIV infection. In spite of these claims, reliable science on ginseng is too meager to support any medicinal benefits (Vogler, Pittler, and Ernst 1999).

The principle active ingredients are called *ginsenosides*, of which thirteen different types are known. Many other compounds, such as sugar, fats, B vitamins, minerals, and phyto hormones (plant hormones), are also present. Another problem with using ginseng is a lack of quality control. Of several dozen commercial products tested, 60 percent had very little ginseng and 25 percent had none at all (Wellness Letter 2000b).

Used in large amounts, ginseng can cause abnormal uterine bleeding, breast soreness, high blood pressure, and ovarian cysts (Scheidermayer 1998; Reichman 1996). Use ginseng with great caution if you have had breast cancer or have high risk factors for endometrial cancer. Large doses over a prolonged period of time provide a significant amount of estrogen, which carries risks for endometrial cancer. Ginseng should not be used with estrogen or corticosteroids (cortisone derivatives) because of the potential additive effects. At present, there is no consistent scientific evidence to support the use of this herb for PMDD.

Dong Quai

Dong quai, sometimes called "female ginseng," has traditionally been used to treat menstrual cramps, menstrual irregularities, and hot flashes. Studies of dong quai used for hot flashes found that it was not more effective than a placebo (Qi-bing, Jing-yi, and Bo 1991). You should avoid it if you have heavy menstrual periods, fibroids, or diarrhea since it can exacerbate these problems.

Other Factors to Consider

If you are considering a future pregnancy, it may be important to avoid echinacea, St. John's wort, saw palmetto, and gingko biloba, all of which have been variously recommended for PMDD/PMS. Under laboratory conditions, all have been shown to adversely affect conception in hamsters, preventing penetration of the egg by sperm (Ondrizek 1999).

Herbs and surgery don't mix. Gingko biloba, ginseng, garlic, feverfew, and ginger have anti-clotting properties that can lead to excessive bleeding. St. John's wort and kava kava (a relaxant) may prolong the sedating effects of anesthesia. The American Society of Anesthesiologists recommends you stop taking all herbs at least 2 weeks before elective surgery (Women's HealthSource 2000).

Homeopathic Treatment of PMDD

The premise of homeopathy is that the mind and body are inseparable and mutually dependent. Homeopathic therapy involves the administration of miniscule doses of substances, which in a healthy person are capable of producing symptoms like those of the condition being treated. Symptoms are regarded as a signal that something has changed and that the mind/body is trying to heal itself. For example, fever is a symptom of infection, and a mood change is a response to an external or internal stress. In homeopathy, symptoms are regarded as more important than the disease process that may be producing them. For this reason, homeopathy is not used for disease prevention.

It is helpful to compare the underlying goals, or philosophies, of different medical disciplines. The goal of traditional Western medicine is to identify and eliminate the cause of illness. Chinese medicine seeks to strengthen the body's ability to deal with disease by harmonizing its energy forces. Homeopathy tries to provoke the body to strengthen its vital forces and heal itself.

Very little is published about effective treatment of PMDD using homeopathic methods. Advocates feel homeopathy should be successful since PMDD is a multisystem disorder and homeopathy addresses the physical, mental, and emotional origins of disease. Since a major tenet of homeopathic treatment is "like is cured by like," meaning the symptoms are first exaggerated if the treatment choice is correct, one wonders how a woman with PMDD would tolerate the early phases of therapy.

All the substances used occur naturally in plants or animals. The following are a few that could be candidates for premenstrual symptoms.

- **Sepia:** This substance is derived from the secretions of the cuttlefish. It is one of the most commonly used homeopathic remedies for fatigue and irritability (Ullman 1991).

- **Evening primrose oil:** The fatty acids of this oil are thought to develop a more effective cell membrane for diffusion of metabolic products, and this is said to improve function of the brain, adrenal glands, eyes, and reproductive organs (Ullman 1991). Evening primrose oil is also used to treat menstrual cramps and premenstrual symptoms. However, as mentioned earlier in this chapter, several placebo-controlled studies have shown that it has no beneficial effect on PMDD/PMS except for relief of breast tenderness.

- **Lachesis:** This substance is derived from the poisonous venom of the American bushmaster snake. The venom is highly diluted and has no toxic effects. Candidates for treatment with lachesis are characterized by homeopathic practitioners as overbearing, demanding, inclined toward fits of rage, and possessing strong libidos (Ullman 1991).

- **Nux vomica:** Made from the poison nut, nux vomica helps nausea, backache, disrupted sleep, perfectionistic tendencies, and chronic anger (Ullman 1991). It is said to help women who are classified by homeopathic practitioners as pushy, impatient, and intolerant types.

- **Pulsatilla:** Comes from the windflower. The "pulsatilla type" is said to be women who are shy, nonassertive, weep easily, have low energy, and low sexual desire. They are usually emotional and needy, wanting lots of attention and comforting.

Naturopathy

The basic philosophy of naturopathy is taken from Hippocrates: "The body heals itself, and the task of the physician is to support this inherent healing potential." Naturopathy involves six basic principles:

1. **Respect the healing power of nature:** The practitioner's responsibility is to remove the impediments to healing and bolster the body's inherent capability to heal itself.

2. **Treat the whole person:** Wellness is a result of the interactions of physical, mental, emotional, spiritual, and genetic factors, as well as environmental, social, and other lifestyle factors.

3. **Do no harm.**

4. **Use the least invasive treatment that will help.**

5. **Identify and treat the cause of illness:** This includes not simply causative agents such as bacteria but also other factors, such as lifestyle, dietary habits, and emotional states.

6. **Prevention is the best cure.**

Naturopaths see their role as educating their patients and encouraging personal responsibility. They use any number of methods, including clinical nutrition, therapeutic manipulation, massage, herbal medicine, homeopathy, and psychological counseling. In Germany, naturopathic services have been found so cost-effective that traditional physicians and pharmacists are required to receive education in naturopathy and botanical medicine (Collinge 1996).

So naturopaths take the best of many disciplines and treat the whole person. The symptoms of PMDD/PMS are as challenging to naturopathic physicians as to any other discipline.

Traditional Chinese Medicine (TCM)

A basic tenet of Chinese medicine is that good health requires that you remain in harmony with the world around you. It is believed that your body is divided into five energy centers, controlled by five organs: kidneys, lungs, liver, heart, and spleen. In classical theory, a life force called Qi (pronounced "chee") flows from one control center to the next, in twelve channels. The channels are like meridians that intersect to form a mesh-like pattern all over your body. More recent theory is that fifty-nine energy channels exist (Fugh-Berman 1997). If the flow of Qi is too much or too little in any channel, an imbalance is created in the network, which in turn increases your risk of disease. A finite amount of Qi exists in your body. It can be depleted by various problems in life, but Qi can also be restored by the use of herbs, diet, acupuncture, and relaxation techniques.

In addition to Qi, there are two other major components of humans: blood and moisture. In order to determine the cause of illness, a TCM practitioner looks for imbalances in moisture/dryness, cold/heat, and excess/deficiency of the three main components, Qi, blood, and moisture, in each of the five organ networks: kidneys, lungs, liver, heart, and spleen. Treatment utilizes herbs, acupuncture, acupressure, and physical exercises such as *t'ai chi* and *qigong* to promote health.

The yin and yang relationship is another concept fundamental to understanding energy balance. Yin and yang are opposite but balancing energies that are present in your body, and for that matter, throughout the universe. If one is at a low level, the other fills in the void and reestablishes the balance by becoming higher. Yin is feminine, and represents things that are cold, dark, still, and heavy. Yang is masculine, and is associated with things that are light, hot, and mobile. A chill is yin and a fever is yang. Low energy is yin, and hyperactivity is yang.

PMDD/PMS symptoms are considered a kidney deficiency in yin energy. Since Qi flows from your kidneys to your liver, you also get a liver-yin deficiency. Now you have a yang excess in both energy centers as opposing balance is restored. Yin deficiency causes insomnia and poor sleep. Liver Qi is associated with anger, so a yang excess here causes rising emotions and irritability. Anger and irritability in turn cause stagnation of liver Qi, which results in distention and bloating (Bienfield and Korngold 1991). To correct this, practitioners use a variety of Chinese herbs, singly or in combination as a tea or an extract. Acupuncture is considered helpful because it is believed to restore the normal flow of energy so the body can heal itself (Lark 1993).

If you decide to try TCM, do so under the guidance of an experienced practitioner. Most states do not require a license to practice, so ask about the practitioner's training and for references from other patients.

Ayurvedic Medicine

According to this ancient discipline from India, all female disorders, including PMDD/PMS are caused by imbalances that fall into three categories: the doshas (body energies), biological rhythm, and body purification. Treatments address these areas of body health. The individual is responsible for self-help through dietary and lifestyle changes. The practitioner's responsibility is to provide the diagnosis and set the appropriate direction of self-care, and also provide herbs to balance the interactions of the doshas (Goldberg 1999).

Balance of the Three Doshas, or Bodily Energies

Vata energy. An imbalance of this type of energy results in mood swings, a tendency to cry, anxiety, and insomnia. Ring any bells? To correct the imbalance, you establish regular daily routines, increase rest and sleep, reduce workload, meditate, and add to your diet more oil, complex carbohydrates, cereal, and warm foods.

Pitta energy. This energy is responsible for female hormone changes. An imbalance results in anger, irritability, skin rashes, and diarrhea. Correction involves reducing overactivity and overperformance, establishing regular daily routines, meditating, and avoiding chocolate, caffeine, alcohol, and fatty foods.

Kapha energy. An imbalance in this energy involves the contents of menstrual flow. It manifests as fluid retention, swollen breasts, weight gain, and lethargy. To correct the imbalance, you must increase exercise, avoid sweets, and increase spicy foods and legumes.

Biological Rhythm

To balance your circadian animal rhythm for darkness and light, it is recommended that you go to bed by 10 P.M. and rise by 6 A.M. This is believed to be the schedule at which the earth's energy enhances human energy.

Purification

This is a concept that menstruation removes *ama* (waste and impurity) from the body. This is facilitated by drinking plenty of water, and avoiding meat, cheese, caffeine, and alcohol.

Craniosacral Therapy

Craniosacral therapy manipulates the bones of the skull to treat a range of conditions, from chronic severe headache to spinal cord injuries, autism, tinnitus (ringing in the ears), and mood disorders. The premise is that there is a rhythmic motion in the cerebrospinal fluid that bathes your brain and spinal cord from your head to the base of your spine. The motion is a wavelike activity that occurs in about six to ten cycles per minute, and is for the most part unaffected by heart and respiratory rhythms.

Craniosacral therapists are trained to recognize the craniosacral motion by gently touching your head and feeling the effects of the rise and fall of cerebrospinal fluid pressure with their hands. In this manner, it is said they are able to detect points of restriction in the fluid's flow which they feel are the causes of the symptoms being experienced. By manipulating the bones of the skull, these restrictions are relieved, normal flow is restored, and nerve tissue becomes healthier.

Premenstrual migraine headaches, common in PMDD sufferers, are said to be relieved in the majority of women who receive craniosacral therapy, and the effect is long-lasting. Treatment of PMDD mood shifts is effective, but this is a short-term benefit.

No controlled studies on craniosacral therapy have been published.

Areas Where Botanical (Plant) Therapies Must Improve

With increasing use of botanicals, it's our opinion that the general public's interests would be better served if a number of problems were addressed.

- More good science is needed, meaning randomized controlled trials published in peer-reviewed journals.

- Study results are hampered by the inability to conduct trials of "single" therapies. By their nature, herbs are complex, containing many nutritional and pharmacological compounds, which are often unpredictable. Researchers should make an effort to identify individual ingredients and study them both singly and in combination.

- Standardization of product preparation by industry suppliers must improve. The current system is inadequate because the botanical product industry is unregulated and not required to prove either safety or effectiveness. A technology exists that can identify herbal ingredients and standardize the products marketed. High performance liquid chromatography (HPLC) can produce an image which demonstrates not only the key components in a botanical but also the relative proportions (Milan 2001). HPLC results do appear on the labels of some products, which implies reliability; but use of this method is not currently required, so most manufacturers omit it.

- The Good Manufacturing Practices (GMPs) label, as required for foods, is not currently being applied to food supplements. The FDA is working with the herbal industry to establish GMPs, so the quality and reliability of botanical products will be improved (Bayne 2000).

- Data on dangers of herbal remedies and adverse drug interactions is lacking. Special problems with herbs are related to growing conditions, plant parts used, and processing.

- The public belief that "If it is natural, it is safe" is often untrue and unsafe.

- Traditional and integrative health practitioners must acknowledge each other. Mutual mistrust results in people becoming reluctant to inform their health advisor of ongoing therapy by another practitioner of a different discipline. This leads to unintended interactions between therapies.

Areas Where Integrative (Alternative) Therapies Must Improve

Since integrative therapies are popular with women who have PMDD/PMS, a systematic review of these methods was carried out by English investigators to determine whether the use of such therapies is supported by valid and rigorous clinical trials. The researchers reviewed twenty-seven studies of randomized, controlled trials (the most reliable science) from seven databases and checked the reference lists of supporting articles. The disciplines studied included herbal medicine, homeopathy, dietary supplements, relaxation techniques, massage therapy, reflexology, chiropractic, and biofeedback. Positive results were acknowledged, but most of the trials suffered from such significant study design flaws that the reviewers were forced to conclude that there is no compelling evidence suggesting that these integrative medical therapies can be recommended for PMDD/PMS (Stevinson and Adzard 2001). This doesn't mean that these therapies are not useful; it simply implies that the advocates of many integrative disciplines have not proven their case with valid scientific studies.

Integrative (alternative) medical disciplines are less well established by credible science for their effectiveness in improving PMDD/PMS symptoms, but there is a rich anecdotal (case-by-case) history of their being helpful. Continued and improved objective study will elucidate the usefulness of these therapies, but at present the clinical value of most remains a murky issue.

PART 3

Medical Interventions

Most people who study PMDD agree that nonmedical self-help approaches should be the initial recommendation for controlling symptoms. Candidates for third party help are women whose symptoms are quite severe or for whom self-help measures failed to provide adequate relief. We urge you not to be discouraged or self-critical if the behavioral changes covered so far in this book have not helped. For some women it's just that way. In chapter 6 we cover the various medications being used for specific symptoms, as well as hormonal treatment. In chapters 7 and 8 we discuss the positive roles that stress management and cognitive behavioral therapy can play. In chapter 9, we explain how to deal with the simultaneous occurrence of PMDD with another mood disorder such as depression or anxiety disorder.

CHAPTER 6

Medications That May Help

Drug treatment for premenstrual symptoms has evolved over the past twenty years, but the most effective drugs have come into use only in the past decade. The general categories are drugs for mood-related symptoms and those for physical symptoms. We will cover the benefits and risks of antidepressant drugs including selective serotonin-reuptake inhibitors (SSRIs) and tricyclic antidepressants. The usefulness of anxiolytic (anti-anxiety) drugs is also discussed. We cover hormonal therapies as well as the uses of diuretics, nonsteroidal anti-inflammatory drugs, and menstrual migraine treatment.

Selective Serotonin Reuptake Inhibitors (SSRIs)

As explained in chapter 2, SSRIs are drugs that prevent serotonin, a neurotransmitter, from being taken back into nerve cells after it has been released for facilitating transmission of a nerve impulse. Serotonin helps regulate moods, sleep, and appetite. Preventing reuptake of serotonin maintains adequate circulating brain levels so that a calming effect occurs. This is why SSRIs work in PMDD.

Most physicians who prescribe SSRIs for PMDD consider them an effective first-line treatment for women who predominantly suffer with mood symptoms. Many placebo-controlled studies have confirmed the efficacy of SSRIs in controlling the emotional symptoms of PMDD (Su, Schmidt, and Danaceau 1997; Ericksson et al. 1995; Yonkers et al. 1997). A positive response to these drugs occurs in over 60 to 70 percent of women (Eriksson 1999). SSRIs currently marketed include fluoxetine (Sarafem, Prozac), paroxetine (Paxil), sertraline (Zoloft), fluvoxamine (Luvox), and citalopram (Celexa).

Another drug that may hold some promise is nefazodone (Serzone) (Freeman, Rickels, and Sondheimer 1994). It inhibits reuptake of both serotonin and norepinephrine, so it acts as an antidepressant. But its effectiveness in controlling PMDD symptoms has not yet been studied.

At this time, fluoxetine is the only SSRI officially approved by the FDA for treatment of PMDD. All of these SSRIs have been used without formal FDA approval for this purpose for many years, however.

How SSRIs Work

Fluoxetine, widely known as Prozac, was the first SSRI available. It has been used successfully since the late 1980s for depression, anxiety disorders, panic attacks, post-traumatic stress, and eating disorders. All of the above conditions have been shown to be associated with low circulating levels of serotonin. Widely sensationalized reports in the media and on the Internet of an increased risk of homicidal or suicidal behavior associated with fluoxetine have been refuted in well-controlled studies (Warshaw and Keller 1996).

Fluoxetine, and all SSRIs, exert their beneficial effect by targeting serotonin selectively, whereas older antidepressants have an effect not only on serotonin but on several other neurotransmitters as well. The older antidepressants spray their target like a shotgun blast, whereas SSRIs have greater accuracy, like a rifle shot. Thus, it is not surprising that a greater array of unintended side effects is more common with the older drugs.

Serotonin has at least six different types of receptor sites in your brain cells. Think of serotonin as a key, and a receptor site as the lock, which can only be entered by a serotonin molecule. Each of these six types of sites receives a specific subtype of serotonin that is capable of influencing different parts of the brain. Some of them control mood, some regulate appetite, and others influence sleep. While serotonin is contained inside nerve cells, it is inactive. The activity is initiated when serotonin is released from nerve cells into the general circulation and then attaches to its various target receptor sites, from which it influences brain cell functioning in specific ways. SSRI molecules resemble serotonin molecules so closely that they can be taken up by nerve cells, which prevents the reuptake of serotonin and in turn raises the circulating level of serotonin available for influencing moods. Since much is yet to be learned about how serotonin exerts its various effects, current research is being directed toward determining the function of each of these six receptor site types. A new generation of SSRIs is being developed that will be able to attach to only those receptor sites that influence PMDD or depressive symptoms. Citalopram, marketed under the trade name Celexa, is one of these drugs. It has the same usefulness as other SSRIs in treating PMDD symptoms, without the associated sexual side effects (Pallanti and Koran 1999). (See the following section on SSRI side effects.)

When it was revealed that PMDD is associated with low brain levels of serotonin, clinical studies of fluoxetine and the other SSRIs was an obvious next step. As you now know, the studies showed dramatic improvement in PMDD symptoms for about 60 to 70 percent. People who look at the cup as only half full point out that 30 to 40 percent are not helped. Why is that? We don't know yet, but it suggests that other causative factors are involved. The additional negative observation is that about 25 percent of women are helped by a placebo, suggesting that an SSRI helps only 35 to 45 percent, not 60 to 70 percent. To the naysayers we say, if 60 to 70 percent say it helps, it helps 60 to 70 percent.

Once fluoxetine was shown to help PMDD, the manufacturer of Prozac applied to the FDA for a new license to market fluoxetine under the trade name Sarafem. (You may remember the Sarafem media blitz that was conducted after FDA approval was granted in 1999.) Some have attributed the reason for this move to the desire to avoid the stigma attached to taking a drug widely used for mental illness. Same medication, just a new name.

But What about SSRI Side Effects?

Fluoxetine and other SSRIs can cause nausea and insomnia in the first few days for about 10 to 15 percent, but this is self-limiting for most. Insomnia can be diminished by taking SSRIs in the morning (Mortola and Moossazadeh 1991). Other problems are agitation, anxiety, shakiness, headache, and sexual dysfunction. Most of these side effects decrease over time (Barnhart, Freeman, and Sondheimer 1995).

Diminished sexual desire and fewer orgasms occur in one-third to two-thirds of SSRI users (Modell et al. 1997). The average is about 40 percent. Since heightened sexual desire is one of the few good things that may happen with PMDD, obliterating it with a drug seems a high price to pay. This is less likely to happen if you take an SSRI only in the luteal (premenstrual) phase instead of every day of the month. Sexual dysfunction is also dose-related and may disappear with adjusting the amount you take. Switching to another SSRI may help. As previously mentioned, Citalopram (Celexa) is an SSRI that was developed to treat PMDD without sexual side effects, and it works (Pallanti and Koran 1999). The addition of buproprion (Wellbutrin) can eliminate sexual side effects of SSRIs (Labbate and Pollack 1994). Sildenafil (Viagra) has been successful in restoring sexual function in women who are SSRI users (Fava et al. 1998). The older tricyclic antidepressants like imiprimine (Tofranil) and amitriptyline (Elavil) do not have sexual side effects, but they don't help PMDD symptoms very well either (Freeman et al. 1999). Look over table 6.1 for a listing of additional SSRI side effects and the percent of women who suffer from them.

A problem with fluoxetine, as opposed to other SSRIs, is its longer half-life (the time it takes for a drug in your bloodstream to decrease by half of the original dose). Fluoxetine's half-life is about a week; traces of the drug can be detected for up to six weeks. The half-life of other SSRIs is about a day. If there is an adverse response to fluoxetine, it could last up to six weeks after you stop taking it, as compared to a week or two with other SSRIs. A benefit of this longer half-life is that there are no withdrawal symptoms if you stop taking it.

Table 6.1   SSRI Side Effects

Type	Number of Women Affected
Sexual dysfunction	35 to 67 percent
Nausea	21 percent
Headache	20 percent
Insomnia	10 to 15 percent
Loose stools	12 percent
Drowsiness	12 percent
Loss of appetite Anxiety Dizziness Tremor Dry mouth	Fewer than 10 percent
Fatigue Constipation Sinus congestion Hyperactivity Blurred vision Cough	Fewer than 5 percent

For PMDD treatment, SSRIs work much faster (usually a day or two) than they do when used for depression and other mood disorders (two to three weeks) (Eriksson 1999). Taking them only during the premenstrual phase turns out to work better for PMDD symptoms than taking these drugs on a continuous basis (Jermain et al. 1999). This is thought to be due to the development of drug tolerance (Eriksson 1999).

Precautions in Using SSRIs

- **Chronic liver or kidney disease:** SSRIs are metabolized in the liver and flushed out when you urinate. If you have serious problems in either your liver or kidneys, SSRIs could build up toxic levels in your blood.

- **History of epilepsy or seizures:** Get a neurological evaluation before starting fluoxetine or other SSRIs.

- **Bipolar disorder:** Because SSRIs may act as a stimulant, they can exaggerate the manic phase in people with manic-depressive (bipolar) disorder.

- **Monoamine oxidase inhibitors (MAOIs):** It is very dangerous to take fluoxetine with MAOI antidepressants (Nardil, Marplan, Parnate). The combination can be fatal. At least two weeks should pass after stopping a MAOI before starting fluoxetine or other SSRIs, and five to six weeks after stopping fluoxetine (two weeks for other SSRIs) before a MAOI is started.

- **Tricyclic antidepressants:** SSRIs enhance the effect of these antidepressants, making it more likely that you would experience insomnia, nausea, loss of appetite, and anxiety. The combination increases the risk of heart rhythm abnormalities and seizure, which are already associated with tricyclics.

- **Antianxiety drugs:** The rate at which your body breaks down these drugs (Valium, Xanax) is slowed by fluoxetine and other SSRIs, meaning the drug will stay in your body a longer time. This is not a serious problem, but it is well to know this and adjust the dose appropriately.

There have been many positive studies reporting the effectiveness of SSRI antidepressants in treating the mood symptoms of PMDD, and most physicians who prescribe them consider them the treatment of choice. In spite of this, surveys have shown that only a very small number of women with PMDD are using SSRIs to combat symptoms. Nonpsychiatrist physicians instead generally offer birth control pills or prescription pain medications.

The Older Antidepressants

Tricyclic antidepressants (Tofranil, Elavil, Anafranil) and monoamine oxidase inhibitors (Nardil, Marplan, Parnate) have been useful for depressive mood disorders for many people. Because they are not particularly selective in the neurotransmitters they target, unpleasant side effects are very common. Weight gain of up to 30 pounds occurs for some users. These drugs are less useful than SSRIs in treating PMDD because they do not enhance serotonin levels nearly as well.

Anxiolytics

Antianxiety drugs may be helpful for PMDD *if* your most prominent symptoms are anxiety and irritability (Harrison, Endicott, and Nee 1990). The most common of these drugs are the benzodiazepines. Alprazolam (Xanax) is the most frequently recommended of the benzodiazepines, but others you may have heard about are lorazepam (Ativan) and diazepam (Valium). The American College of Obstetricians and Gynecologists (ACOG) recommends reserving these medications for women whose symptoms have not been relieved by other interventions (ACOG 2000).

An advantage of benzodiazepines is that they're fast-acting. Unfortunately, it's also easy to develop a tolerance, which can lead to larger doses, and drug dependence. To minimize this risk of addiction, these drugs should be used only in the premenstrual phase of the cycle. Side effects include drowsiness and lightheadedness. Therefore they are best taken before bedtime.

Hormonal Treatment of PMDD

For more than thirty years, researchers and clinicians have thought that abnormal blood level variations of estrogen and progesterone were in some way the source of the 100 to 150 premenstrual symptoms that plague so many women. Over these years, all sorts of attempts at hormonal cure-alls have met with only checkered success. Each one claimed to eliminate or favorably modify the wide array of annoying to life-altering symptoms associated with PMDD. Meanwhile, research has shown that PMDD/PMS occurs almost exclusively in normal hormonal cycles (Rubinow 1992). These observations confirmed that PMDD/PMS is an abnormal response to normal hormonal production.

Progesterone—Can It Help Control PMDD?

In short, progesterone does *not* help control PMDD. In the early to mid-1980s, however, it would have been heresy to say that progesterone therapy had no effect on what was then known exclusively as PMS. Natural progesterone vaginal suppositories were the main treatment for premenstrual symptoms throughout the 1980s. When studies showed that the 80 percent effectiveness of natural progesterone suppositories was essentially the same as placebo suppositories, enthusiasm for this treatment waned rapidly (Mortola 1992). In addition, no differences in benefits could be demonstrated between high or low doses of the vaginal progesterone (Freeman, Rickels, and Sondheimer 1990). Among the other 20 percent of women studied, neither the placebo nor the progesterone had any effect (Epperson, Wisner, and Yamamoto 1999). In a separate study it was further demonstrated that progesterone blood levels were the same in women suffering from PMDD/PMS and those who were not (Schmidt, Grover, and Rubinow 1993).

There are still devotees of natural progesterone cures, but they are hopelessly behind the times. Progesterone does not seem to help women with PMDD except in cases of breast pain and tenderness, where it was show to be significantly more effective than a placebo (DiCarlo et al. 1997).

Micronized Natural Progesterone Creams

Progesterone creams, made from micronized (pulverized) natural progesterone, are being widely advocated for treatment of premenstrual symptoms. When rubbed into the skin, they are absorbed directly into the bloodstream. You start using the cream mid-cycle, right after ovulation, and continue using it until your menstrual period begins. Although there are some PMDD sufferers who are enthusiastic about progesterone cream, when these creams were tested against a placebo there was no difference. Don't be fooled by the claims that these creams will help—they won't (Smith and Schiff 1993; Epperson, Wisner, and Yamamoto 1999; Huston and Lanka 2001).

Estrogen May Help

Many premenopausal women in their forties use an estrogen skin patch to alleviate anxiety, migraine headaches, and negative moods associated with PMDD/PMS. Researchers believe that estrogen is not a cure for most premenstrual symptoms, but it does cure certain symptoms that may start during the premenopausal years (the five or so years before menopause) (Revlin, Morrison, and Bates 1990; Leventhal 1996). They feel that premenopausal PMDD/PMS is really due to a late luteal phase decline in estrogen levels. Extra estrogen (by either skin patch or pill) during the week to ten days before your period is due will usually relieve anxiety, menstrual migraines, and other negative feelings associated with PMDD/PMS. Unfortunately, it won't reduce bloating, breast soreness, or menstrual cramps, and your menstrual flow may get a little heavier.

Apply the patch once you begin to experience premenstrual symptoms. Place it away from your breasts and away from skin creases. The estrogen will begin to work within an hour.

If your PMDD/PMS symptoms are very predictable every month, you may want to take oral estrogen, such as low-dose estradiol (Estrace), rather than use the skin patch. To relieve your symptoms, you take it every day beginning seven to ten days before the expected date of your menstrual period.

Oral Contraceptives (OCs)

Because OCs suppress ovulation and hormone production by your ovaries, a combination OC (estrogen + progestin) or a progestin-only OC may relieve premenstrual symptoms. Reports on the efficacy of OCs for PMDD/PMS have been inconsistent, with some reporting improvement and others reporting that symptoms get worse (DiCarlo et al. 1997).

The American College of Obstetricians and Gynecologists suggests OCs if the premenstrual symptoms are primarily physical (ACOG 2000). Triphasic OCs, in which the levels of estrogen and progestin vary throughout the month, were initially thought to be more effective in alleviating the physical symptoms than monophasic OCs, in which estrogen and progestin levels stay the same (Backstrom et al. 1992). More recent opinion is that the monophasic pill is better (Huston and Lanka 2001).

A new OC is being studied that shows promise for treating PMDD. It contains a new type of progestin called *drospirenone*. The FDA approved it in 2001 to be marketed under the trade name *Yasmin*. Yasmin is monophasic, which is thought to be more effective for controlling moodiness (Brown 2001). In addition, drospirenone has a diuretic effect that prevents premenstrual fluid retention, and it is antiandrogenic, meaning it blocks male hormone. This latter effect diminishes mood swings and reduces acne.

Adverse effects of an OC trial include nausea, breakthrough bleeding, breast tenderness, and headache. They are contraindicated if you have had *deep-vein thrombosis* (blood clots), undiagnosed abnormal uterine bleeding, or an estrogen-dependent tumor as with some breast cancers. OCs are also contraindicated if you are a smoker over the age of 35, because of the increased risk of heart attack (Medical Economics Company 2000).

Thyroid Hormone

In the 1980s, there was some belief that PMDD/PMS was a result of hypothyroidism. The studies that suggested this were shown to be flawed, and later studies indicated thyroid hormone treatment was no more effective than a placebo (Nicolai, Mulligan, and Gribble 1990). If hypothyroidism is suspected, it should be diagnosed and treated first. If premenstrual symptoms persist, you may need other treatment.

Stop the Ovaries and You Stop PMDD

If you don't ovulate, you don't have PMDD. Interfering with ovulation is a radical approach that we don't advocate unless PMDD symptoms are very severe, and other treatments have failed. It isn't difficult to block the ovaries from functioning, but the cure may be worse than the disorder, due to long-term side effects. Nevertheless, as a last resort, you may want to consider the following techniques.

GnRH Agonists

GnRH agonists are synthetic chemicals that shut down your ovaries. GnRH means gonadotropin-releasing hormone. Gonadotropins are hormones produced in the pituitary gland (FSH and LH) that target the gonads (ovaries) and stimulate them to function. A GnRH agonist overstimulates and eventually blocks this activity. It essentially produces a chemical menopause that is effective in controlling PMDD symptoms (DiCarlo et al. 1997). For women with depression or other mood disorders, GnRH agonists are less helpful (Freeman et al. 1993).

You can take GnRH agonists by injection (leuprolide; Lupron), as a nasal spray (nafarelin; Synarel), or in the form of subcutaneous pellets (goserelin; Zolodex). After the initial dose, a temporary outpouring of FSH and LH by the pituitary may aggravate and intensify PMDD symptoms in the first two to three weeks. Estrogen production eventually drops, however, and a false menopause occurs. The PMDD symptoms may be gone, but you may experience hot flashes, short-term memory deficits, sleep disruption, vaginal dryness, and mild mood swings (Huston and Lanka 2001). The menopausal symptoms can be relieved somewhat by "add-back" therapy with low doses of estrogen, but it is not as effective for PMDD relief as when GnRH agonists are used alone (Leather et al. 1999).

Long-term side effects of this artificial menopause include loss of bone mineral density, which raises the risk for future osteoporosis, plus increased risk for heart disease. For these reasons, GnRH agonist therapy is not recommended for longer than six months (Mortola 1997). GnRH agonists are also expensive.

Danocrine

Danocrine (marketed as Danazol) is a weak synthetic androgen (male hormone derivative) that is helpful in relieving mental and physical PMDD symptoms (Mortola 1997). It acts on the pituitary and hypothalamus to inhibit secretion of FSH and LH, so that ovarian function and menstrual periods stop.

Because danocrine halts ovarian function, there are significant side effects, some of them rather similar to premenstrual symptoms. They include depression, weight gain, and bloating. Loss of estrogen may cause hot flashes, vaginal dryness, and moodiness. In addition, the fact that danocrine is a male hormone derivative may also cause decreased breast size, acne, excess hair growth, and deepening of the voice. Some of these changes may become permanent, especially a deepened voice. Long-term use can adversely affect your cholesterol profile, decrease bone density, and accelerate cardiovascular disease (Mortola 1994). Based on the risk-benefit ratio, danocrine is not a good choice for treatment of PMDD.

Ovariectomy

Surgical removal of the ovaries relieves PMDD symptoms completely (Casson et al. 1990). However, it subjects you to immediate menopause with all of the related symptoms plus the long-term health threats of estrogen depletion (osteoporosis, cardiovascular disease). Estrogen can be replaced, but if you are under age forty, it is difficult to keep estrogen at a high enough level with hormone replacement. Therefore, ovarian removal should be considered in only the worst cases of PMDD, when nothing else has helped.

Medications for Physical Symptoms

Diuretics

Diuretics are prescription drugs that increase urine production to eliminate the accumulation of excess fluids. The most commonly used diuretic for PMDD is spironolactone (Aldactizide), which can be effective in relieving premenstrual fluid retention, weight gain, and breast tenderness (Wang, Hammarback, and Backstrom 1995). Potassium depletion is a problem with long-term or frequent use of most diuretics, but not with spironolactone. Loss of potassium can lead to heart rhythm abnormalities. Other diuretics such as hydrochlorothiazide (Esidrix, HydroDiuril) and furosemide (Lasix) can be used if spironolactone is ineffective.

Diuretics tend to be effective for premenstrual symptoms only in women who gain weight. Diuretic abuse is common in women who are overly concerned with their weight (Mortola 1994). "Water pills" should not be regarded as harmless medications. Over dosage can lead to nausea, vomiting, diarrhea, drowsiness, dizziness, and mental confusion.

Nonprescription Drugs

Nonsteroidal inflammatory drugs (NSAIDs). These are effective for treatment of menstrual cramps, premenstrual cramps, and headache. Ibuprofen (Motrin) and naproxen (Naprosyn) are among the most widely used over-the-counter medications for premenstrual symptoms (Singh et al. 1998). Uterine contractions (cramps) during a menstrual period are caused by chemicals called prostaglandins. When it was discovered that NSAIDs are antiprostaglandins, they became quite popular. An old study of naproxen found it to be effective if taken twice daily starting seven days before menstrual flow and continuing for a few days into the period (Facchinetti et al. 1989). Premenstrual moods improved, which seemed to result from pain relief. (**Caution:** If used over a prolonged time, NSAIDs can cause stomach upset or an ulcer, and may lead to kidney problems in the elderly and in diabetics.)

Acetaminophen. This is a widely used drug for self-treatment of premenstrual symptoms. Pamprin, Premsyn, and Midol contain acetaminophen, as well as parabrom (a diuretic) and pyrilamine (an antihistamine). Their manufacturers claim they relieve such premenstrual symptoms as irritability, tension, headache, backache, cramps, bloating, and water weight. Although these products have been available for many years, no well-controlled scientific studies have confirmed their effectiveness (Moline and Zendell 1997).

Menstrual Migraines

Menstrual migraines are severe headaches occurring a few days before your menstrual period is due, or during the first few days of flow. Headaches are commonly preceded by difficulty concentrating, a mood change, or a food craving. About 15 percent of migraine sufferers experience an "aura" just before the headache begins. Symptoms during the aura can include a particular smell, flashing lights, numbness, or tingling. Following the aura, a pounding, throbbing headache begins. Other symptoms include nausea, vomiting, and photophobia (sensitivity to light). Most women who have menstrual migraines seek out a dark, quiet place to lie down. Migraines may be severe enough to keep you home for a couple of days. The special distinction of *menstrual* migraines, of course, is that they occur once a month.

Tension headaches are also a common PMDD symptom, so it helps to be able to distinguish between the two types. Table 6.2 illustrates how they differ.

Table 6.2 Characteristics Differentiating Migraines from Tension Headaches		
Characteristics	**Migraine Headaches**	**Tension Headaches**
Location	One or both sides	Both sides
Frequency	Intermittent	Intermittent
Duration	8 hours (2–72 hours)	Variable
Pain	Throbbing (50%)	Often band-like
Severity	Moderate to severe	Mild to moderate
Associated symptoms	Nausea, vomiting, photophobia	Uncommon
Family history	Often present	Present

Adapted from: S. D. Silberstein. 1990. "Advance in Understanding the Pathology of Headaches." *Neurology.* 42 (2):6–10.

Prevention of Menstrual Migraines

A number of medications can help prevent migraines.

- **Estrogen:** Menstrual migraine is thought to result from the normal drop in estrogen just before your period begins. Some women avoid this drop and prevent a migraine with an estrogen skin patch applied daily one week before their period is due. Estradiol, an oral estrogen, also works.

- **SSRIs:** Serotonin is known to be low during any type migraine attack. Selective serotonin reuptake inhibitors (Sarafem or Prozac, Zoloft, Paxil, Luvox, Celexa) may help with migraines. If you have PMDD and a regular monthly migraine, a luteal phase SSRI may prevent your migraine attacks.

- **NSAIDs:** The anti-prostaglandin effect of NSAIDs, mentioned earlier in this chapter, can prevent menstrual migraines. NSAIDs should be taken every six to eight hours for a week before your period is due and into the first two or three days of menstruation.

- **Prevention with testosterone:** The use of testosterone pellets injected beneath the skin may help (Lanka and Klingman 1997). The testosterone from the pellet goes directly into the bloodstream, and gets converted into estrogen in the woman's brain (Leventhal 1997). This increased estrogen level in the brain and the resulting higher serotonin level may explain its effectiveness.

- **Danocrine (Danazol):** Because of its androgenic properties, danocrine can be effective in preventing menstrual migraines, but the side effect profile of this drug (mentioned earlier) makes it less than a top choice.

- **Calcium:** One study found that women who consume the recommended daily amounts of calcium (1,200 mg) and vitamin D (400 IU) have fewer menstrual migraines (Thys-Jacobs 1994).

Treatment of Menstrual Migraines

If you can't prevent your migraines, you can treat them.

- **Ergot alkaloids:** These commonly employed blood vessel constrictor drugs have been in use for many years for migraines. Ergotamine and dihydroergotamine (DHE) are effective in stopping the onset of a migraine *if* taken at the very first sign of an attack. A self-administered injection of DHE at the critical time works well for most, with a second dose an hour later if no relief is experienced. Only two shots can be used in a twenty-four-hour period. DHE is also available in tablet, nasal spray, lozenge, aerosol, and suppository form.

- **Triptan drugs:** These are relatively new drugs that successfully treat migraine attacks by masquerading as serotonin. They attach to serotonin receptor sites and prevent serotonin reuptake, which makes for higher brain levels of the neurotransmitter, and effective treatment. Unlike the ergot alkaloids, triptan drugs can successfully relieve a migraine even if not given at the outset of an attack. You can take them by injection (self-administered), in pill form, or by nasal spray. Several are now available: sumatriptan (Imitrex), zolmitriptan (Zomig), rizatriptan (Maxalt), and naratriptan (Amerge). Because triptan injections can cause a heart spasm, you should try it for the first time in a hospital setting.

- **Integrative (alternative) medical therapies:** Alternative medical therapies can be remarkably effective in reducing migraine pain. You may want to consider them, especially if you've been plagued by the side effects of drug treatment. Biofeedback and acupuncture work quite well for many women. Both are good for stress reduction, and stress is a well-known migraine trigger. Hypnotherapy, massage therapy, osteopathic manipulation and craniosacral therapy can also be effective in moderating migraine pain.

Drug treatment can be quite successful in relieving the life-altering symptoms of PMDD. The treatments covered in this chapter are not for everyone, of course, but it should be comforting to know that an armamentarium of effective and well-researched treatment is available if you need to employ it. It's true that access to these therapies requires third party help in the form of your health advisor, but advice from a knowledgeable source can also be valuable. The next chapter focuses on managing stress, a major contributor to PMDD.

CHAPTER 7

Stress: A PMDD Culprit

Women who suffer from PMDD are more likely to have ongoing problems with stress. As we explained in chapter 2, there are biological reasons why women with PMDD have an abnormally high response to stress. As yet, it isn't clear what can be done to favorably alter this abnormal stress response, but there are many methods for dealing with the stress that you may have. If you learn to control the stress itself, you can help control your PMDD. This chapter will define stress, explain what it does to you, and suggest a variety of methods for managing the stressful events that confront you.

A Definition of Stress

Stress isn't easy to define, but one generally accepted description is that stress is the sum of your biological reactions to any adverse stimulus that disrupts your homeostasis, or balanced state. Homeostasis is a constantly changing balance in the physiological, psychological, and social spheres of your life. It functions in a series of ongoing minor adjustments that will usually bring you back into balance when stress has thrown you off kilter. The adverse stimulus can be physical, such as fatigue from insomnia; it can be mental, as when you can't maintain your concentration; or it can be an emotion, as with fear.

The stimulus causing stress is called a *stressor*. It is any change arising externally or internally, whether real or imagined, that requires you to react or adapt to it. Not everyone reacts the same way, of course. If your reaction to a stressor is inadequate or inappropriate, it can lead to a variety of stress symptoms and many other problems.

Stress-Related Problems

Infectious diseases of various sorts have always been the predominant cause of illness and death over the centuries, but stress-induced disease has now assumed this mantle in industrialized cultures (Notelovitz and Tonnessen 1993). Stress is linked to heart disease, asthma, arthritis, chronic pain, infertility, insomnia, cancer, depression, and now PMDD. There is solid evidence that stressors such as anxiety, loneliness, grief, negative emotions, and depression will suppress your immune system (Kiecolt-Glaser and Glaser 1991; Kiecolt-Glaser 1996). A suppressed immune system puts you at risk for a variety of illnesses, including the common cold, as well as a failure to respond to protective vaccines.

Each time you are confronted by a stressful or threatening situation, your brain instructs your nervous system to rapidly release stress hormones into your bloodstream. Each time, your body reacts because a stressor is something that threatens your physical or psychological well-being. The magnitude of the threat (and therefore the stress) depends on whether you feel you can cope with it. Most of the stresses we face don't require coping techniques like a primal scream with fists balled or a hasty retreat from the scene. This fight-or-flight reaction is hard on your body and your health, which is why it's important to find ways to control your responses to stress.

Stress responses have more significance for you as a woman than for men because stress hormones stay in your bloodstream longer (Harvard Women's Health Watch 1999). Because stress hormones suppress your immune system, you are more at risk for infectious diseases and other illnesses if such episodes are frequent or chronic. You can control the damage, however, by recognizing stress and coping with it more effectively.

Recognizing Stress

Sometimes the symptoms of stress are easier to recognize than the source. The symptoms may be emotional, physical, behavioral, or cognitive, and you may sometimes have symptoms in all of these categories. Table 7.1 lists some typical symptoms.

The source of stress is sometimes obvious, such as a relationship going awry, a job change, or loss of a family member. Some aren't so obvious. If your hair is turning gray, if you suddenly need reading glasses, if you notice new wrinkles, you might not recognize any one of them as a

Table 7.1   Symptoms of Stress

Emotional	Physical	Behavioral	Cognitive
Anxiety	Rapid heart rate	Critical of others	Forgetfulness
Nervousness	Restlessness	Can't get things done	Can't make decisions
Anger, acute or chronic	Headaches	Bossy with others	Fuzzy thinking
Irritability	Stomachaches	Overeating	Diminished creativity
Loneliness	Insomnia	Excess smoking	Lost sense of humor
Boredom with life	Sweaty palms	Overuse of alcohol	Constant worrying
Feeling pressured	Fatigue	Neglect of personal habits	Trouble concentrating
Fearfulness	Breathlessness	Decreased sexual desire	
Crying	Tension, neck and shoulders		
Unexplained sadness			

stressor. If you nevertheless feel stressed without other apparent causes, it could be that the aging process itself is the stressor for you. Finding the source on your own can be difficult, and you may want to seek expert help from a psychological counselor. Whatever the cause of your stress, once you identify it, you are in a much better position to effectively deal with it. (Chapter 8 covers some therapies that may help you locate your sources of stress.)

Dealing with Stress

People who adapt to stress more naturally than others are said to have "stress-hardy" personalities (Kobasa, Maddi, and Kahn 1982). Such individuals are able to experience stress without undergoing the typical adverse physical and/or mental stress responses. Stress-hardy people seem to share some important traits:

1. They tend to accept challenges.

2. They have a sense of control over life's capriciousness.

3. They are committed to their families, to their work, and to life in general.

Instead of passively accepting life's vagaries, stress-hardy people tend to take control of situations. They are more likely to regard challenges as opportunities for personal growth than as threats to be avoided. When confronted with a stressful situation, people with stress-hardy personalities confront it, explore the possibilities the conflict presents, and get involved in problem-solving. People who have a weak response to stress tend to react to stress more passively, with an attitude of helplessness. Most of us fall somewhere between these two extremes.

Stress-hardy individuals tend to form close personal relationships (Benson and Stuart 1993). They are able to both provide and receive social support. People who are isolated tend to be less stress-resistant.

Wherever you fall on the stress-hardiness curve, you can improve your response to stress. Stress doesn't need to have a negative impact on you; you can turn it to your advantage. Your *reaction to stress* is what governs its effect on your life, your health, and the severity of your PMDD. Your goal should be to reduce heavily stressful influences in your life as much as you can and to learn better coping strategies. Don't adopt a strategy of avoiding stress entirely; you simply won't succeed. Instead of regarding stress in largely negative terms, though, you can try to perceive it as a stimulus to achievement. Actively coping with stress challenges your intellect and engages your emotions. Indeed, you may achieve a more desirable result by changing your reaction to a stressful situation than by changing the situation itself.

Strategies for Coping with Stress

Effective coping is dependent on a number of factors:

- healthy diet
- adequate exercise
- psychological adjustments that produce a positive attitude
- relaxation techniques

Psychologically, you have a number of built-in defense mechanisms that help in moments of stress. These automatic mental maneuvers temper the intensity of your emotional reaction to a stressful situation (Huston and Lanka 2001). Good coping utilizes mature defenses, and poor coping uses immature defenses. A mature defense to missing seven straight traffic lights would be a quiet resignation that you will be a little late. An immature defense would be pounding your fist on the steering wheel while shouting obscenities and driving recklessly. The long-term problem of poor coping is that it can aggravate your PMDD and lead to a number of social maladjustments, such as chronic anger and estrangement.

Your built-in defense mechanisms help you counteract the everyday, simple stresses of life: when you can't find your car keys, your child's little league team just lost, or you have incinerated the family dinner. You may handle these stresses without even noticing how you did it. When the stresses are extreme (as when a family member dies) or long-lasting (you are diagnosed with a threatening disease), they can overwhelm you, and their effects can become harmful to your health and aggravate your PMDD. There are many ways you can reduce the negative impact of stress.

Eat a Healthful Diet

If you are under considerable stress, you may be too distracted to focus on your nutritional needs. But good nutrition is more important than ever because stress raises your metabolic rate and increases your energy needs. A diet emphasizing complex carbohydrates that are high in fiber is known to be beneficial for PMDD because of the calming effect from increased serotonin (discussed in chapter 3). It works for stress control as well.

Get Regular Exercise

Aerobic exercise is a dependable method of reducing stress. Brisk walking, cycling, step-aerobics, and swimming are all beneficial because they provide a useful outlet for your fight-or-flight energy. Endorphins are released into your circulation during vigorous exercise. They elevate your mood, and produce a state of natural relaxation. Your blood pressure declines, your pulse rate decreases, your muscles become relaxed, and tension is released. Exercise during the day helps you sleep better and your mind will benefit from the general relaxation. You should exercise daily, or even twice daily, for about thirty minutes, to get the best results. It doesn't need to be two trips to the health club every day. A couple of brisk walks will do nicely. Note: Refrain from exercising before bedtime; you may become overstimulated, which can prevent sleep.

Get Plenty of Rest

Insomnia is a common accompaniment to stress and PMDD. Insomnia causes chronic fatigue, which in itself can be an additional stressor. Prescription sleeping pills can provide relief in acute situations, but many are too addicting for long-term treatment. In addition, they become less effective with continued use. You can also become dependent on over-the-counter sleeping aids, so try to avoid that path as well. Improving your sleeping habits is your best long-term option. Consider the following recommendations for helping you sleep (Benson and Stuart 1993):

- **Spend less time in bed:** The average adult needs only seven to seven and a half hours of sleep (Hauri and Linde 1990). This Mayo Clinic study showed that spending too much time in bed is the most common mistake you can make if you have problems with insomnia.

- **Eat a light carbohydrate snack an hour or two before bed:** A snack such as cookies or cereal may help to increase your production of serotonin, the brain chemical that promotes sleep.

- **Control your sleeping room:** It should be dark, quiet, and reasonably cool. Pull the shades, wear eye covers, and use ear plugs if necessary to manage your sleeping environment.

- **Maintain a sleeping schedule:** Try to establish a sleeping rhythm by going to bed at the same time every day and getting up at the same time. Your body will accommodate to your schedule.

- **Avoid caffeine late in the day:** Coffee, tea, and cola soft drinks are the chief suppliers of this stimulant.

- **Use your bed exclusively for sleep:** Except for having sex, of course. Don't eat, watch TV, talk on the phone, or work in bed.

Make Psychological Adjustments

There are a number of things you can do to become better adjusted psychologically for confronting stress.

Look for Social Support

PMDD may be considerably accentuated when major life stresses confront you. If infidelity, divorce, work dislocation, children leaving home, financial problems, or single parenthood are on your plate, you may benefit from joining a group of women who are facing similar problems. Talking about your stresses and sharing your feelings with others who are experiencing similar disruptions in their lives can reduce stress significantly. Support groups for various health and personal concerns can be found in most communities. You can find them through newspaper listings or the yellow pages of the phone book, community hospitals, religious organizations, or mental health clinics, or by word of mouth.

Prioritize the "Shoulds" That You Face

Sometimes an accumulation of little things that you need to do are annoying and represent the stressor. Some people call these tasks "shoulds." Individually, they aren't much, but as a group they can be stressful. They may have been piling up for weeks or months, or maybe the list just started yesterday. In dealing with your "shoulds," try ranking them according to their priority:

1. Essential

2. Important

3. Trivial

A good way to assign rank is to ask yourself: "What is the worst thing that could happen if I don't get this done?" You'll find that many tasks you first thought were crucial or essential just aren't. You may find you want to downgrade many items on your list of "essential things that I should do immediately" to "what the heck" after you have subjected them to the "what is the worst thing that could happen?" test. Then concentrate on the remaining essential items, see if you can't recruit some assistance on completing the important tasks, and ignore the trivial stuff (Landau, Cyre, and Moutlon 1994).

When assigning priorities to your list, be sure to include some time for yourself near the top of your "essential" column. Even if it is for only a few minutes, plan something that pleases you and is just for you. Simple pleasures like luxuriating in a warm bath or reading a passage in an inspirational book do nicely. Or try reading the daily messages of comfort and joy that Sarah Ban Breathnach presents in *Simple Abundance*. She details six principles of simple abundance and how they blend to help you find the authentic life you were born to live (Breathnach 1995).

Avoid the Quick Fix

Many health care professionals and their patients rely on the prescription drug route for managing stress. Our "instant relief" society has been conditioned to expect a "pill cure" from tranquilizers, and antidepressants. These drugs do indeed have usefulness in acutely stressful situations, but drug therapy tends to deal with symptoms only. It fails to address the underlying causes of severe stresses and the importance of taking responsibility for dealing with them. The same may be said for alcohol use during stress. The National Institute of Alcohol Abuse and Alcoholism has stated that if you consume alcohol during stress, you become more intoxicated and experience a worse hangover than when you use it during more relaxed periods. And lighting up a cigarette to relax is counterproductive because nicotine releases epinephrine, the very stress hormone you already have circulating in abundance. Use of street drugs also falls into the category of temporary avoidance.

Learn How to Relax

The kind of relaxation we are talking about is much more than a leisurely stroll, or going to a movie. For stress management, a large number of special relaxation techniques are available to you. Deep breathing is one

of the simplest, yet effective relaxation methods. Others include meditation, progressive muscle relaxation, visualization and guided imagery,
self-hypnosis, biofeedback, laughter, religion, yoga, t'ai chi, massage, acupuncture, and acupressure. The goal of all of these methods is to elicit the
"relaxation response" (Benson and Stuart 1993). This is a state of con-
sciousness during which you have diminished your skeletal muscle tension, oxygen consumption, breathing rate, heart rate, blood pressure, and
even your skin's electrical conductivity. This is the opposite of what happens in your body during a fight-or-flight stress response. As a matter of
fact, when you have successfully elicited the relaxation response, it is
impossible to feel fear or anxiety (McKay, Davis, and Fanning 1997). When
practiced regularly, these techniques are effective in reducing general,
interpersonal, and performance anxiety, all of which are experienced in
PMDD.

Deep Breathing

Deep breathing is one of the most widely used methods of relaxation.
It is often used as the starting point for other techniques, such as meditation, yoga, and visualization. The following exercise elicits the relaxation
response (McKay, Davis, and Fanning 1997):

- Seat yourself comfortably in a quiet room and close your eyes.

- Relax all of your muscle groups by consciously thinking of each of
  them one at a time. (See section on progressive muscle relaxation.)

- Breathe in slowly and out slowly through your nose, and concentrate on the air you are moving both into and out of your body.

- Repeat a word or phrase silently. Any neutral word—one that
  does not provoke anxious thoughts—will do. For example: peace,
  tranquility, contentment. Such repetition will help to keep extrane-
  ous thoughts out of your mind.

- Allow about ten to fifteen minutes to do this.

- At the end, sit quietly for another minute or two before slowly
  opening your eyes.

Abdominal Breathing

The purpose of abdominal breathing is to relax the muscles of your
abdominal wall. In stressful situations, they tighten and put pressure
against your diaphragm. This limits how far your diaphragm can descend
to pull air into your lungs. The net result is shallow breathing, which can
make you feel as if you are not getting enough oxygen and lead to

hyperventilation and panic. When you are feeling stressed, it may only take three or four deep abdominal breaths to produce effective relaxation.

Try the following exercise (McKay, Davis, and Fanning 1997):

1. Lie down and close your eyes. Put one hand on your chest and the other on your abdomen just below your waist. As you breathe in, imagine you are sending the air as deeply into your body as possible. When you do this, the hand on your chest will move somewhat, but the hand on your abdomen will rise and fall much more with each breath.

2. If the hand on your abdomen doesn't move much, press it lightly against your abdomen as you inhale and attempt to push it up as you breathe in deeply.

3. Once you've mastered the technique, continue to gently breathe in and out at whatever pace seems natural. Then start counting each exhalation until you reach ten, then start over. Continue to do this for about ten minutes.

Progressive Muscle Relaxation

This is an effective means to relax when anxiety and fear have resulted in your storing tension in your muscles. It has long been known that tension can be released by firmly tightening your muscles for a few seconds and then relaxing them suddenly and completely (Jacobsen 1974).

We've adapted the following exercises to help you with your PMDD. These exercises involve four major muscle groups: arms, head, torso, and legs. If you do them twenty to thirty minutes daily, or ten to fifteen minutes twice daily, you can produce the relaxation response you seek. As you do them, tighten each muscle group for seven seconds and relax for twenty seconds. Notice carefully what your muscles feel like during the relaxation phase. This will teach you the physical signs of relaxation, which is key to recognizing the relaxation response (McKay, Davis, and Fanning 1997).

1. **Arms Exercise**
   - Clench both hands into fists and hold them for seven seconds as tightly as possible without straining, then let go suddenly and relax for twenty seconds. Repeat.
   - Bend both elbows and flex your biceps for seven seconds. Relax suddenly and focus on the sensations of relaxation. Repeat.
   - Tighten your triceps by locking your elbows and straightening both arms by your sides for seven seconds. Relax and focus on the sensations. Repeat.

2. Head Exercise

- Wrinkle your forehead by raising your eyebrows as high as you can for seven seconds. Let your eyebrows drop suddenly. Relax for twenty seconds. Repeat.

- Scrunch your face as if you are trying to make your entire face meet at the tip of your nose. Relax for twenty seconds. Be aware of the feeling during and after the contraction. Repeat.

- Clamp your eyes tightly closed and smile as widely as you can. Hold for seven seconds and relax for twenty seconds. Repeat.

- Clench your jaw muscles and push your tongue against the roof of your mouth. Hold for seven seconds and relax for twenty seconds. Repeat.

- Open your mouth into a large "O." Hold, relax, and repeat.

- Tilt your head back as far as it will go. Hold, relax, and repeat. Tilt your head toward one shoulder for the same routine. Then roll your head to the other shoulder. Return your head to its normal position and feel the tension ebbing away. Stretch your head forward until it is resting on your chest, and feel the tension release as you return to the normal position. Repeat.

3. Torso Exercise

- Raise your shoulders toward your ears, hold them in this position for seven seconds, and release. Relax for twenty seconds. Repeat. Stretch your shoulders back like you are trying for your shoulder blades to touch. Let your arms drop to your sides. Relax and repeat. Pay attention to the heavy feeling in your muscles as you relax.

- Position both arms straight out from your shoulders. Cross one over the other as high up on your arms as possible and hold. This stretches your upper back. Feel the tension release when you let your arms drop to your sides. Repeat.

- Take a deep breath and hold it while tightening all the muscles in your abdominal wall. Exhale and release the tension. Repeat.

- While sitting or lying down, gently arch your back. Hold this position for seven seconds, then relax so your back flattens against your chair or the floor. Repeat.

4. Legs Exercise

- Tighten your thighs and buttocks. Increase the tension by straightening your legs and pushing down toward your heels. Hold seven seconds. Relax for twenty seconds, and repeat.

- Press your legs together as hard as you can to tense your inner thigh muscles. Hold, relax, and repeat.
- Tighten your leg muscles while pointing your toes away from you. Hold, relax, and repeat.
- Draw your toes upward to tighten the muscles of your calves. Hold, relax, and repeat.

Find a place where you can have some quiet and solitude to do your progressive muscle relaxation routine. Be sure to allow enough free time to get through the exercise. You can add to its effectiveness if you start with slow, deep breathing as described previously.

After you know the routine, you can shorten it somewhat by doing several of the recommended exercises simultaneously. Tighten all the muscles in your arms at the same time. While doing the head rolls, scrunch your face muscles, too. While pointing your toes away from you, tighten your thighs and buttocks as well.

Once you become familiar enough with what relaxation feels like, you can pick out the areas of your body that are tense by scanning the four areas of the basic exercise. You can simply "let go" as you have become accustomed to doing after tensing your muscles. You can also learn to relax your muscles on cue whenever you want by combining a verbal suggestion with abdominal breathing. On each inhalation of abdominal breathing, simply say the words *breathe in*, and on exhalation say *relax* while letting go of tension throughout your body. This teaches your body to associate the word *relax* with the feeling of relaxation. After a while you will be able to achieve relaxation just by mentally repeating *breathe in . . . relax* (McKay, Davis, and Fanning 1997).

Transcendental Meditation

Meditation is a well-known alternative in relieving a wide variety of ailments, including stress. Meditation utilizes deep breathing, already described. In addition, it often involves repeating a mantra (word or phrase) and incorporates a variety of additional relaxation methods. You can do it sitting or lying down, while enjoying a peaceful walk, or even during other forms of exercise.

Meditation involves learning to have a quiet inner self and to live more actively in the moment. It can help you become more alert and energetic, and more serene. Getting started requires some training, so if you're interested, look for a beginner's class at your local mental health clinic, community center, or church.

If you decide to try meditation, make a commitment of several months. Over time doing meditation can have a positive effect on you, lowering your levels of stress and relieving your PMDD.

Visualization and Guided Imagery

With visualization, you fill your mind with a relaxing image in order to help you relax. You mentally construct a peaceful scene in a setting that is appealing and in which you feel safe and secure.

Start with the deep breathing exercise we've already described, close your eyes and focus on an image of utter serenity or profound joy. Think of a past event in your life that made you feel good. Maybe it was a certain sunset, maybe your wedding. Involve all of your senses in the image you are creating in your mind. Think about every detail of the event: the time of day it happened, the surroundings, who was there, what was said, what you were wearing, how it felt, how it smelled, what you were feeling. Return to this peaceful scene if you are having a PMDD day and feeling stressed. It's fun to do and exquisitely relaxing.

If focusing on an actual event doesn't work for you, guided imagery may help. This involves listening to a someone, either in person or on tape, narrate a scene for you, to help you create an image of serenity in your mind.

Hypnosis can also be used as a form of guided imagery. It is a safe and effective means of relaxing; but it requires the help of someone specifically trained. You can also learn to relax using self-hypnosis.

Biofeedback

Biofeedback uses various recording devices to monitor heart rate, blood pressure, and skin responses, in order to teach you to identify tension in your body. When you are tense, the recordings are dramatically different from when you are relaxed. Using visualization, guided imagery, and other relaxation techniques, you can monitor whether, and how much, your tension is being relieved.

Yoga

Yoga is a system of physical exercises, postures, and stretching combined with deep breathing that requires you to focus on your body. As a woman with PMDD, you may discover that yoga is not just a wonderful way to relax but also a way to improve flexibility in your body. It is probably a good idea to start with a class to learn the basics. Look for yoga classes at your local community college, fitness club, or on videotape.

T'ai Chi

T'ai chi is a discipline of exercise and breathing that originated in China. It means "Salute to the Sun" and Asians traditionally use it to greet the new day. T'ai chi emphasizes breathing, body alignment, and flexibility, which makes it similar to yoga. The difference is that the techniques of t'ai chi are designed to stimulate your body as well as to relax it, which is why it is an effective way to start your PMDD day. T'ai chi is becoming increasingly popular in the U.S., so look for announcements and ads for local classes, if you're interested.

Acupuncture

Acupuncture is an ancient Chinese technique for treating many health problems, and it works for stress as well. Tiny needles are inserted at specific locations to positively alter the flow of energy, called Qi (pronounced "chee"). Many people find it works to advance healing and promote overall well-being. It can also induce relaxation in PMDD sufferers. The benefit you receive is dependent upon the skill of the practitioner, so be sure you see a licensed acupuncturist. (Acupressure, a similar technique, applies pressure, but not needles, to the appropriate locations.)

Laughter

Humor relieves stress both psychologically and physiologically. Everyone knows there's nothing like a good laugh to relieve a tense situation. Laughter relaxes your muscles, puts more oxygen into your system, and lowers blood pressure, not to mention it has a unique ability to defuse a confrontation. As Victor Borge observed: "Humor is the shortest distance between two people." When you're having one of your grim PMDD days, humor can help you cope. You may have to look pretty hard for something funny on those days, but usually there is a thread of humor somewhere. Keep a scrapbook of really great jokes or cartoons you've found in newspapers and magazines and review it when you feel PMDD taking control of you. Go to funny movies during PMDD; the laughter of an audience can be infectious. Just listening to how different people laugh is funny in itself!

A sense of humor is like a first-aid kit that you carry with you at all times. It is available at a moment's notice to improve your mood, defuse a confrontation, lower your blood pressure, and relieve your anxiety. Here is a five-point plan for improving your life with laughter, adapted from a lecture on how laughter can improve your health (Wilde 1997). We've adapted some of these points to specifically address your problems with PMDD.

- **Laugh out loud:** Physically laughing, as opposed to just grinning or thinking about laughing, increases oxygen in your system, improves your circulation, lowers your blood pressure, and even has a positive influence on your immune system.

- **Laugh at yourself:** At its roots, laughter is an expression of love. If you can laugh at your own shortcomings, especially during PMDD, you basically like yourself and you have healthy self-esteem. Abraham Lincoln, never known as a handsome man, had this comment when he was accused by someone of being two-faced: "If I had two faces, would I be showing you this one?" Abe was comfortable with himself.

- **Maintain a lighthearted attitude:** Only you are responsible for your attitude. You can choose your attitude toward any situation, even with PMDD. If you choose to make it upbeat, stress control will be easier, resentments will be defused, and you'll even be a more productive worker.

- **Find something funny every day:** Some days you may have to dig pretty deep to find something funny; life is like that. Maybe it will be only a cartoon in the newspaper, but find something.

- **Find the funny side of life even when you are suffering from your PMDD:** You might as well laugh instead of cry. When everything has seemingly turned against you, it is not inappropriate to resort to humor. A famous humorist once wrote that just as life does not cease to be funny when we have a serious problem, life does not cease to be serious when we laugh.

Laughter is good for you and your PMDD. It doesn't cost a dime; it's tax-free, fat-free, cholesterol-free, and nontoxic. As humorist Josh Billings said: "There ain't much fun in medicine, but there's a heck of a lot of medicine in fun."

Religion

Many people benefit from a commitment to a formal religion and a deeply felt set of values and beliefs. Religious traditions and beliefs can provide a sense of depth and meaning in life. Thus, a commitment to religion can help you in developing an awareness of a larger reality and promote an understanding that life has meaning and significance (Moyers 1993). The peace you derive from this kind of awareness is a good antidote for stress.

Massage Therapy

Therapeutic massage can be an extremely pleasurable and relaxing experience. Massage therapists can be usually found at beauty salons and health clubs. Mutual massage is a good option, and you can get some tips on therapeutic massage from a video or book on massage. In addition to its relaxing benefits, massage can provide an affectionate and romantic interlude for you and your partner. Facials can also be very relaxing when done professionally.

Hot Tubs and Saunas

Hot tubs and saunas feel great after a workout, or if you just wish to relax during the PMDD era of your cycle. Usually, about fifteen minutes in water around a hundred degrees is all it takes. After exercising, however, you should avoid water or a sauna that is too hot; it can divert too much blood from your central circulation and cause you to faint. If you have not cooled down after exercise or you have just consumed a large meal (which concentrates blood in your abdomen for digestion), plunging into a hot tub or entering a sauna can lower your blood pressure enough to make you faint. As a precaution, enjoy a hot tub or sauna with someone else. It's more fun anyway.

Psychotherapy

Short-term therapy is yet another method of handling stress. This is less structured than most of the above techniques, and it is more personalized. A major goal of stress management is to first identify the stressor. In many instances the underlying source of stress is obscure, and you may need some counseling to help identify it.

Effective management of stress is an important adjunct to controlling PMDD. This chapter has presented a variety of ways to cope with stress. Not all of them will work for you, of course, but you may find several of them beneficial. In the next chapter we cover cognitive behavioral therapy (CBT), which is yet another very helpful means of dealing with PMDD.

CHAPTER 8

Cognitive Behavioral Therapy

Cognitive behavioral therapy (CBT) has been a successful psychological treatment for mood disorders such as depression and anxiety for about forty years (Ellis 1962). Cognition refers to thinking, perceiving, and remembering. Thus, cognitive behavioral therapy refers to treatment focused on how your thoughts influence your feelings and emotions. This makes sense because how you think about any given situation determines your feelings. Positive, negative, or neutral thoughts result in corresponding feelings, for example, happy, sad, or nonplussed.

Since a hallmark of premenstrual dysphoric disorder is severe mood change, it stands to reason that CBT should be helpful. Studies have shown this to be the case (Koons 1999; Davis and Yonkers 1997; Kirkby 1994). In this chapter, we will introduce a case study to show how two kinds of cognitive therapies work. The goal of these therapies is to help you identify errors in your thinking that lead to negative moods. Learning and utilizing some of the techniques discussed may help you control your PMDD.

Nancy's Story

Nancy is a forty-year-old woman who came in for therapy because she was feeling "hopeless, helpless, angry, and scared much of the time." She was afraid that her marriage was in trouble because of her anger and depression. Nancy has been married to Ed for fifteen years, they have two children ages thirteen and ten, and Nancy describes her marriage as "her rock." She states that she and Ed agree about so many things, especially how to raise the children. However, the one area she and Ed constantly argue about is money. Nancy describes herself as a "saver" and Ed as a "spender." They are well-off financially, but she lives in fear that they will not have enough.

For the past ten years Nancy has been feeling sad a good deal of the time. She describes herself as "pretty easygoing and fun most of the time." However, Nancy relates an almost continual monthly pattern of feeling sad and angry for about ten days prior to the onset of her period. She has described what she says is "wicked PMS." Her PMS symptoms include bloating, salt and chocolate cravings, plus fatigue, sleeplessness, irritability, and muscle tension. All of these symptoms go away, along with her feelings of sadness and anger about two days after her period starts. She has worked with her medical doctor to help her with her PMS; however, both she and her physician believe that Nancy may be experiencing something more than just PMS.

Initially her therapist had Nancy keep a diary of her feelings, thoughts, and behaviors. Her therapist asked her to write out a chart using a calendar of the days of her menstrual cycle and her moods, thoughts, and behaviors for each day of the month. After two months of charting, it became clear that Nancy's feelings of depression and anxiety were related to her menstrual cycle. Nancy said that just knowing these feelings were somehow related to her periods helped her to feel less hopeless and helpless. "Since there is a biological reason for a lot of my feelings, I guess I don't feel like this bitchiness is just a part of my personality that will last forever."

Nancy was very interested in cognitive behavioral therapy as a tool to help her with her PMDD. She continued to see her Ob/Gyn for medication and did a great deal of cognitive work to help her handle her symptoms. As we discuss a couple of different models of cognitive behavioral therapy, we will use Nancy's case as an example of how they work.

How Cognitive Behavioral Therapy Works

All of us exist within a very complicated environment. We are affected by what is happening within our bodies on a chemical level. We are affected by what happens at work and within our families. We are affected by traffic on the freeway and the food we choose to eat. We are affected by air and water pollution and by political events, such as what is happening in the Middle East.

Our thoughts (cognitions), feelings (emotions), biology (hormones and predisposing medical conditions), behaviors and environments (families, friends, finances) all affect how we feel. They are all interconnected. Think of them as five parts of a mobile. When you touch one part all the other parts move and shift to balance out the changes made by the part you touched. For example, when we exercise, our bodies release endorphins that make us feel good, which helps us to think positively about ourselves, which in turn makes us more receptive to and able to handle things at work and at home.

Because of these interconnections, our thoughts can play a huge role in maintaining negative feelings of depression, anger, and anxiety. For example, when Nancy first came in for therapy she was feeling very sad and hopeless. On the calendar where she was charting her thoughts, feelings, and menstrual cycle, she wrote down her thoughts as: "I am sick." "There is something really, really wrong with me." "I will never feel better." "I can't do it." "It's too hard." Repeat Nancy's thoughts out loud and ask yourself what it must feel like to be thinking those thoughts.

In therapy, Nancy learned to identify her negative thoughts, evaluate whether these thoughts had merit, and change her dysfunctional or irrational thinking patterns so that her mood improved.

Types of Cognitive Behavioral Therapy

There are several models of cognitive behavioral therapy of which two models are the most widely researched and used. The first is Albert Ellis's *rational emotive therapy* (Ellis 1999).

Although PMDD is very similar to depression, it should be easier to treat. Because you know that a lot of your negative feelings are associated with normal changes in hormone levels related to your menstrual cycle, you can predict the timing of these feelings. Then, because you can predict when these negative feelings may arise, you can use some effective cognitive behavioral tools to help prevent and treat those negative feelings. To effectively treat PMDD you need to build skills to help identify, test, challenge, and change your irrational beliefs and negative automatic thoughts.

Rational Emotive Therapy

Albert Ellis developed rational emotive therapy based on the belief that our problems don't develop from external events but from our *views* or *beliefs* about these events. Emotional distress develops when our beliefs are irrational, a tendency that we all have to some degree.

The ABC Theory

Based on the above, Ellis developed the ABC theory of cognitive-behavior therapy (1962):

A is an Activating event

B is an irrational Belief about A

C is a Consequence of the belief

D is a necessary Dispute (or challenge) to B so that

E the Effect of the irrational belief will not persist

Let's look at how the first three of these components interacted in Nancy's case.

A is an activating event, behavior, feeling or attitude. As an example, Nancy and Ed have always made major financial decisions together. During their marriage Nancy has always been the "saver" and Ed has tended to want to splurge and spend their money a bit more freely. They have both worked throughout their marriage, and have made good salaries. Nancy has desired a large retirement savings, large college education savings for their children, and a large "rainy day fund." Bass fishing has been Ed's passion for ten years. He goes fishing at least once a week. Recently Ed bought a new, expensive rod and reel. Nancy became very angry that Ed would go out and spend that much money on a "toy." So, this was the activating event for Nancy.

B is an irrational belief about A. As a consequence of Ed's spending, Nancy became irate that Ed would disrespect her needs and would go back on their agreement to make joint decisions concerning spending large sums of money. She had visions of losing the house, of the kids not being able to go to college, and of Ed and her being homeless after retirement. She became very depressed and anxious.

As you read the above scenario it may appear that **A** caused **C**—that Ed's spending money on a new rod and reel caused Nancy to become angry and depressed. However, Ellis states that **A** does not cause **C**, but that there is a **B**, a belief about **A**, that causes **C**. Nancy may have only felt a little irritated if she had told herself, "It was thoughtless that Ed didn't talk to me first about buying a new rod and reel, but it really wasn't that much money. He works hard and deserves to treat himself to something sometimes. We still have money in savings. We may not be able to add as much money as usual into our saving accounts this month, but we'll be fine." In reality what Nancy told herself was, "He obviously doesn't care about me or the kids. He's selfish and wasteful. All he cares about is himself. He can't be trusted. He should care about our future more than his stupid fishing. He must dedicate himself to the future like I do." Those irrational beliefs cause Nancy to feel anger, outrage, indignation, depression, and resentment.

If Nancy does not challenge or dispute **(D)** her irrational beliefs, then the effect **(E)** will persist and she will remain depressed, angry, hostile, and resentful.

A negative ABC scenario plays out for Nancy during her PMDD episodes. The monthly changes in her hormone levels affect Nancy's ability to tolerate frustration well, and cause her to have stronger negative emotional reactions. Generally Nancy and Ed are very successful at working things out in their relationship. Given the problems the couple has when she is premenstrual, Nancy has found it helpful to use the ABC model.

As with most couples, Nancy and Ed have certain "hot button" issues in their marriage. Money is one of those issues for them. During their marriage they have been fairly successful in learning to compromise and to respect each other's needs concerning money. They have agreed to discuss all purchases that are more than $500 with each other. They have agreed to put a certain amount of money each month into their savings accounts. In response to Nancy's PMDD, they've also agreed to not discuss any major money issues during the ten days prior to Nancy's period.

C is a consequence of the belief. The feelings you have after an activating event depend on whether you experience rational or irrational beliefs about it. The activating event in our example was Ed spending money on a new rod and reel for bass fishing without discussing the purchase with Nancy first. The consequences of Nancy's beliefs will be desirable or not, depending upon what she thinks (Ellis and Bernard 1986). Nancy's beliefs are in quotes in the scenarios that follow.

1. **Desirable emotional consequences:** "Ed has spent money again. He works hard for his money and he deserves to treat himself to something now and then. Fishing makes him so happy. He hasn't gone over our spending limit." Nancy has no negative feelings, or may have warm feelings toward Ed.

2. **Desirable behavioral consequences:** "I know I have a strong need for financial security. Just what impact did Ed's spending that money really have on our future financial security?" Nancy examines their long-range financial goals and decides that they are well on their way to meeting their goals. She and Ed decide that they need to have some fun with some of their money and they decide to give themselves each an allowance that they can spend anyway they wish without needing to consult each other first.

3. **Undesirable emotional consequences:** "Ed spent money again. Ed does not love or respect me. He knows how important money is and yet he doesn't care about me or the kids. He wants us to end up homeless. He's selfish. He should care and understand." Nancy

feels hurt and is overwhelmed by anger, resentment, and depression.

4. **Undesirable behavioral consequences:** "Ed never listens to what I say. He doesn't care about my needs. He should know how important financial security is and he should respect that! He obviously doesn't care." Nancy yells and screams at Ed. He leaves the house to avoid Nancy's yelling. She gets scared and angry, fearing she'll lose Ed, begins to cry, and retreats into her room.

Musturbation Causes Irrational Beliefs

An important underlying premise about irrational beliefs is what Ellis has labeled *musturbation*. Musturbation occurs when your preferences, desires, and wishes become absolute necessities—unconditional "shoulds," "oughts," and "musts." Musturbatory thinking leads to three irrational beliefs (Ellis 1984):

1. **Awfulizing:** "The way Ed spends money we will be penniless and homeless. Our children will not be able to attend college."

2. **Self-damnation:** "If only I was a better and more beautiful person, Ed would love me enough to save money. I must not be important enough to him."

3. **I-can't-stand-it-itis:** "I can't take any more of this disrespect. I'm out of this marriage. He doesn't care about me."

When you become trapped in musturbatory thinking, you will feel angry, depressed, anxious, or any number of other negative emotions. By believing that the world "should be fair and just," that you "must be loved and cared for by everyone," and that people "ought to know what you need," you set yourself up to be disappointed, angry, resentful, and depressed. It's easier to identify and challenge your musturbatory thinking during times when you are not experiencing PMDD. By writing down your musturbatory beliefs and writing down your challenges to those beliefs, you can develop ammunition to fight irrational beliefs before they cause negative emotions.

Challenging Musturbatory Beliefs

In Nancy's case, she decided to challenge her musturbatory beliefs. She divided a sheet of paper into two columns. In one column she wrote down her musturbatory beliefs, in the other column she wrote out challenges to those beliefs.

Belief: "The way Ed spends money we will be homeless and the kids will never get to go to college."

Challenge: Nancy looked over the checkbook and credit card statement for the past six months; and realized that Ed had only spent what was equivalent to his agreed-upon allowance. Some months he spent only a small fraction of his allowance and saved the rest to make a single big purchase after a few months. Nancy spent all of her allowance each month; she had assumed Ed did the same. Nancy realized her mistake in thinking that Ed was overspending.

Before this, Nancy and Ed had met with a financial planner who had helped them establish savings goals for their retirement and the children's college education. Nancy reviewed these goals and realized they were more than meeting their goals each month.

Belief: "If Ed really loved me, he would save money. I must not be loveable or beautiful enough for Ed to really love me."

Challenge: Nancy sat down and made a list of all the loving things Ed had done for her recently. He had washed her car, made her breakfast in bed on her birthday, took her to her favorite restaurant on their anniversary, rubbed her feet when they watched TV, washed and dried the dinner dishes, brought her flowers, and told her he loved her and thought she was beautiful at least every other day.

Belief: "I can't stand any more of this disrespect. I am out of this marriage."

Challenge: Nancy sat down and made a list of the pros and cons of getting a divorce. She had a huge list of cons and could only think of one pro—she would have complete control of her money. Nancy realized that she loved Ed and he loved her and that she didn't want to end the marriage. What she did want was to feel financially secure. She realized by reviewing her financial status that she could feel secure and that Ed was not overspending. Ed's taking care of his needs was not disrespecting her needs. He was able to meet his needs within the defined limits of their agreement and Nancy was able to feel secure within those same limits.

This list became very important to Nancy. She realized that for the most part she really felt secure and loved within her marriage. It was during her PMDD that she became irrational and depressed about money. Nancy referred to this list to help her find balance during her PMDD, which helped her to avoid overreacting to money issues. She decided that before she responded to something that was irritating or frustrating to her, she would read through her lists to decide if she was musturbating.

Nancy also made up a notebook of issues and situations that would trigger her depression, anger, or anxiety during her PMDD. She found that if she identified her irrational or musturbatory thoughts and wrote out rational responses to these thoughts before she experienced her PMDD symptoms, she was quite successful when PMDD arrived. If she tried to do this while experiencing PMDD, she was unsuccessful.

Irrational Beliefs

Ellis and Harper (1979) identified a list of ten common irrational beliefs:

1. You must have the love or approval of all the people you find significant.

2. You must prove thoroughly competent, adequate, and achieving.

3. When people are obnoxious and unfair, they should be blamed and seen as bad, wicked, or rotten.

4. Things are horrible and catastrophic when you get seriously frustrated, treated unfairly, or rejected.

5. Emotional misery comes from external pressures and you have little or no ability to control or change your feelings.

6. If something seems dangerous or fearsome, you must preoccupy yourself with it and make yourself anxious about it.

7. You can more easily avoid facing many of life's difficulties and self-responsibilities than undertake more rewarding forms of self-discipline.

8. Because something in your past once strongly influenced your life, it has to keep determining your feelings today.

9. People and things should turn out better than they do and you must view life as awful if you do not find good solutions to these realities.

10. You can achieve maximum human happiness by inertia or inaction or by passively "enjoying yourself."

As you were reading through this list, did any of these statements make you smile, nod your head, or trigger a statement of "Yeah . . . ?" Again, everybody has irrational beliefs. The goal is to be able to identify those beliefs and to challenge and dispute them so you will not need to suffer the negative consequences. The latter can be anything from feelings of depression to low self-esteem to feelings of dissatisfaction with your relationship, your job, and life in general.

Identifying Irrational Thoughts

Sometimes one of the most difficult parts of cognitive behavioral therapy is to be able to identify your irrational thoughts. You know you are angry and you can't understand why you are reacting so strongly. While the situation that is angering you is irritating and frustrating, you can fully see that your reaction is out of proportion to the situation.

To deal with this, Ellis and Grieger (1977) have made some helpful suggestions for detecting irrational beliefs:

1. Look for "awfulizing" and ask yourself, "What is awful about this situation?"

2. Look for beliefs such as "I can't stand it!" and examine what about the situation is really unbearable.

3. Look for "musturbating" thoughts and determine what "shoulds," "oughts," and/or "musts" you're telling yourself about the situation.

4. Look for blaming or "damning" yourself or others and ask, "What is really unforgivable about this behavior?"

Another simple way of detecting irrational beliefs is to look for them in one of three major "musturbating" categories:

1. "I am worthless unless I always do well and receive complete acceptance." (I *must* be perfect and be loved by everyone.)

2. "People and life should always be fair and kind." (Life *must* be fair and provide me what I deserve.)

3. "If someone really loved me, they would know what I need and want without my needing to tell them." (Love and caring are magical and *must* always be experienced that way.)

Disputing Your Irrational Beliefs

Now that you have learned to identify your irrational thoughts and beliefs, what's next? You need to learn to dispute them. Write out one of your irrational thoughts on a piece of paper or in your journal. Now ask yourself: "What evidence is there to support this belief?"

In Nancy's case she identified one of her irrational beliefs to be: "The way Ed spends money we will be homeless and our children will not be able to attend college." Then she debated the belief.

Support for Nancy's belief:

- Ed just spent a lot of money on a new rod and reel.

- Ed insists we go out to eat at least once a week.

Dispute of Nancy's belief:

- Ed really just saved up his allowances and spent the money on his new rod and reel. He didn't touch our savings account.

- Ed likes nice things, but he doesn't really spend that much money.

- We are able to meet our saving goals every month.

- Even if we were not able to meet our savings goals for a month or two, we would be a long way from being homeless.

By debating this belief, Nancy was able to realize she was overreacting and felt better.

Another way to dispute irrational beliefs is to discriminate between

- wants and needs

- desires and demands

- rational and irrational ideas

- absolute and non-absolute values and behavior.

One of Nancy's irrational beliefs was that she must be perfect and nice all of the time in order for people to love her. In discriminating between this belief and the reality that not everyone could always love and accept her all the time, Nancy realized she had been setting herself up to feel like a failure. By discriminating between rational and irrational ideas, Nancy was able to tell herself, "I'm human and I will make some mistakes and not everyone will always love me. It would be nice if they did, but it is unrealistic to expect them to always love me and that I can be perfect."

Nancy was able to successfully handle her feelings of anger, irritation, depression, and frustration during her PMDD episodes by learning to identify and challenge her irrational beliefs. She realized that she had no control over the situations that confronted her during the ten days of her PMDD episodes, but she did have control over how she chose to react to those situations and events. Nancy created what she called her "PMDD conscience." This was a notebook she used to write out potentially activating situations and events and rational responses and beliefs to those events. Because Nancy was able to plan ahead, she became very successful in coping with her negative moods and reactions during PMDD.

Cognitive Therapy

Since "cognitive" means "to know" or "to think," cognitive therapy is viewed as the psychological treatment of thoughts. It assumes that thoughts, beliefs, attitudes, and perceptual biases influence not only the emotions you experience but also the intensity of those emotions. The therapy teaches you to identify and monitor your negative ways of thinking and negative behavior and then to change those thought and behavior tendencies so that you will function in a more realistic fashion. It takes a fair amount of personal effort and discipline to learn the necessary skills, but if you can use them to control the negative moods of your PMDD, it may well be worth it.

Aaron Beck's cognitive therapy (Beck et al. 1979) is similar to Albert Ellis's rational emotive therapy in that it also focuses on your thoughts and beliefs in the treatment of anxiety and depression. But Beck and other cognitive therapy theorists believe you develop automatic thoughts (which are usually negative when you are depressed) in response to underlying negative assumptions about yourself, the world, and your future. Cognitive therapy focuses on exploring these negative automatic thoughts and underlying assumptions and challenging them in order to create a more balanced and realistic view of yourself, the world, and your future. By creating a more balanced view, your emotions and moods become more balanced and less negative. Through Beck's cognitive therapy Nancy was able to learn more about how her responses to situations and events are based on the way she perceives these situations and events.

Family History and Psychological Disorders

There can be many predisposing factors that influence the development of psychological disorders. A strong family history of a specific disorder is one of them. In such instances, biological factors may predispose you to developing certain psychological disorders. The environment you grew up in also taught you different ways of coping with stresses. For example, if your father handled negative feelings associated with a job he disliked by drinking, you may have learned to numb your negative emotions in the same manner. If your mother handled her negative feelings by becoming withdrawn and depressed, you may assume those same behaviors.

In Nancy's case, her mother and her maternal grandmother both suffered from depression. Because both have passed away, Nancy was unable to determine whether her mother's depression may have been PMDD. Using Beck's theory, we can see that Nancy seemed to have a predisposition toward depression and PMDD, based on her mother and maternal grandmother's histories of depression. Nancy may also feel her marriage, financial security, and future are threatened, which in turn can cause distorted interpretations and perceptions.

Cognitive Distortions

Cognitive distortions are errors we make in reasoning when we are experiencing psychological distress (Beck 1967). These include:

- **Arbitrary inference:** Drawing a specific conclusion without sup-porting evidence or even in the face of contradictory evidence. An example of this would be when Ed spent money on a new rod and reel and Nancy concluded, "Ed spent so much money, now we're going to be homeless and the kids won't be able to go to college."

- **Selective abstraction:** Conceptualizing a situation on the basis of a detail taken out of context, ignoring other information. An exam-ple of this would be when Ed spent his allowance money on a new rod and reel and Nancy concluded, "He doesn't love me."

- **Overgeneralization:** Abstracting a general rule from one or a few isolated incidents and applying it too broadly and to unrelated sit-uations. For example, when Nancy and Ed ended up in a big fight after Ed bought the new rod and reel Nancy concluded, "We have a terrible marriage and will never be able to communicate."

- **Magnification and minimization:** Seeing something as far more significant or less significant than it actually is. An example of this is when Nancy concluded that all of their savings was gone because Ed spent some money. Or when Ed made Nancy breakfast in bed and took her to her favorite restaurant Nancy saw it as nothing much.

- **Personalization:** Attributing external events to oneself without evidence supporting a causal connection. When Ed was taking about how much he wanted a new rod and reel Nancy made a harump sound, but never really told him her feelings. When Ed bought the rod and reel Nancy believed that Ed did it to her delib-erately, and that it was a direct sign that Ed did not care about her, listen to her, or love her.

- **Dichotomous thinking:** Categorizing experiences in one of two extremes, for example seeing yourself as totally successful or a total failure. Or seeing yourself as totally loved or totally hated.

The Cognitive Model of Depression

Beck has described what he calls a cognitive "triad" of depression (Beck 1967). Depressed people will have a negative view of themselves, the world, and their future. They will see themselves as flawed, inadequate, unlovable, and worthless. They will view the world as grey and uninter-esting, threatening, and overwhelming. They will view their future as hopeless.

The goal is to correct what Beck terms "faulty information process-ing" and to modify the assumptions that perpetuate these dysfunctional behaviors and emotions. Applying this idea to PMDD, you would challenge the dysfunctional beliefs that may be creating your PMDD depression, and promote more realistic, balanced thoughts.

Challenging your dysfunctional beliefs is done by viewing them as hypotheses that can be examined and tested. After challenging your beliefs, you will need to decide whether to reject them, modify them, or maintain them.

Defining the Problem

One of the first steps in cognitive therapy is to define the problem. To do this, you should ask yourself some questions about the problem:

- **How is the problem maintained?** Analyze the factors that perpetuate the problem. For example, one of the factors perpetuating Nancy and Ed's disagreement over money was that a discussion about spending a lot of money on new fishing equipment would have taken a long time, so Ed chose not to talk to Nancy about it. Nancy became very angry when he did not talk to her before buying the equipment. This caused a big fight which perpetuated Nancy's feelings of anger and depression.

- **What are the situations in which the problem occurs?** Nancy's anger, anxiety, and depression seemed to happen when she was feeling insecure, or when she felt that Ed wasn't respecting her need for security and control. This was especially true during her PMDD.

- **How frequently do these situations occur?** If, in your case, the problem occurs only once a year, then maybe it is not that much of a problem. But if the problem is occurring once a week or several times a month, then maybe you should be more concerned. Given the subject of this book, of course, you might find it particularly noteworthy if the problem occurs only when you're premenstrual.

- **How intense are your feelings and how long do they last?** While these situations may occur very infrequently, they may be of such intensity that you should focus on them in therapy. Nancy found herself feeling angry, resentful, and depressed for days after a fight with Ed. Because these feelings were so long-lasting she felt it was very important to seek counseling.

- **What are the consequences of the problem?** Nancy's feelings were causing her to push Ed away. Her feelings of anger and resentment were putting a great deal of strain on her relationship. Because the consequences of her feelings of anger, depression, and anxiety were so negative, Nancy decided it was time to seek professional assistance.

The next step is to complete an analysis of the problem:

- What are the thoughts and images you have when an emotion is being triggered?

- What do you imagine will happen in a distressing situation?

- What is the probability of that really happening?

As a part of your analysis, it is very important for you to be able to identify your thoughts and feelings and discriminate between them. While this may sound easy, many people have trouble due to confusing thoughts with emotions. To help you, we've included a list of common feelings at the end of this chapter. It is also useful to write out *thought records*. An example of a thought record is included at the end of the chapter. If you are prone to cognitive distortions, it may also be useful to keep a *thought record*, in which you write down your thoughts when you have strong emotions about a situation. Thought records can be used to help you identify your cognitive distortions and to better understand the emotions you may attach to certain situations or thoughts (Beck et al. 1979). For example, if you find yourself getting angry when your partner leaves the room and refuses to talk to you, is it their leaving or the thoughts you may attach to the situation ("He hates me." "She will never come back." "I'm a total bitch.") that upset you?

You can keep your thought records in the form of a journal. At the end of this chapter, we've given you a sample outline, asking you to describe an upsetting situation, to identify and rate your feelings based on their intensity, to write down your thoughts (which may contain some faulty thinking), to come to a more balanced thought, and then rate your feelings again. This may seem awkward in the beginning, but once you get used to using thought records you will be able to complete them very quickly and to analyze them effectively.

Because your thoughts, emotions, and brain chemicals are fluctuating during your PMDD episode, it is very important that you begin to use thought records *before* you are experiencing PMDD. Nancy found it very helpful to keep a notebook of her thought records; she found that many of her dysfunctional thoughts were repeated over and over again in different situations throughout the month. As Nancy practiced this technique, she was able to identify a pattern of her cognitive distortions and the feelings that arose from these distortions. A big clue to her PMDD reactions was the intensity of her negative feelings. While she had negative thoughts and feelings during other times of the month, the negative thoughts and feelings she experienced during her PMDD episodes were extreme. For example, if Nancy was driving on the freeway and someone cut her off, she routinely became angry. During most of the month Nancy rated her anger about a 5 on a scale of 1 to 10. Her thoughts included, "What a jerk. I can't believe he just did that!" However, if the same thing happened to Nancy on the freeway when she was premenstrual, her anger rose to a 10 on the same scale. Her thoughts became, "That SOB, how dare he do that to me! Who does he think he is? I'll show him!" By recognizing her changed intensity of feelings to similar provocations, Nancy could confirm their origin as PMDD, and cope with them more successfully.

While Beck's cognitive therapy may seem a little more complicated than Ellis's rational emotive therapy, it is highly effective. Nancy found rational emotive therapy to be very effective in helping her to handle her symptoms of PMDD. Still, Nancy chose to move from rational emotive therapy techniques and to focus more on cognitive therapy because she found it to be more effective in helping her understand some of her childhood issues that shaped her dysfunctional thinking.

Traditionally, both rational emotive therapy and cognitive therapy were designed to be used in psychotherapy with professional therapists. We highly recommend that you seek out professional guidance and assistance with your PMDD if at all possible. If you want to get a sense of the techniques of cognitive behavioral therapy, try some of the exercises presented in this chapter. If you find yourself struggling with them or overwhelmed with negative feelings in spite of them, then see a qualified mental health professional trained in cognitive therapy or rational emotive therapy.

Most qualified professionals are able to work on a short-term basis (eight to twelve sessions) with you using cognitive therapy. Your state's psychological association referral service can be an excellent source for locating a licensed professional. Be sure to ask about specific training and experience in working with cognitive behavioral therapy for PMDD. This is important to you, so be specific in stating your needs.

Feelings List

To help you identify your feelings, we've included this list of common feelings, dividing them into five main categories, or emotional states: *mad, sad, glad, scared,* and *ambivalent.* Feel free to add words to describe other feelings that you sometimes have.

Mad: closed, annoyed, cheated, attacked, angry, cold, self-destructive, disgusted, defensive, mean, inconsiderate, irritated, rebellious, aggressive, deprived, enraged, petulant, furious, infuriated, hateful, jealous, envious, cross, offended, manipulated, pissed off, resentful, controlling, self-loathing, smothered, spiteful, greedy, vengeful, suffocated, used, distant, moody, vicious, indignant, exasperated, bitter, violent

Sad: depressed, humiliated, embarrassed, judged, unhappy, unlovable, unloved, hurt, blue, unattractive, disconnected, ashamed, down on yourself, lonely, unappreciated, put-upon, helpless, emotional, bad, dumb/stupid, betrayed, abandoned, rejected, disillusioned, disempowered, weak, shameful, unsupported, despairing, self-pitying, lost, left out, isolated, sorry for yourself, on trial, exploited, powerless, battered, victimized, inferior, dirty, abused

Glad: clear, brave, cared for, centered, happy, connected, content, classy, cuddly, blessed, smart, powerful, attractive, aroused, fulfilled, alive, big, delighted, excited, free, serene, full, flattered, grateful, grounded, heard, honored, saved, satisfied, inspired, creative, strong, loving, mothered, nurtured, peaceful, playful, protected, proud, relieved, safe

Scared: powerless, apprehensive, frightened, anxious, fearful, on guard, excluded, jittery, criticized, crazy, guilty, shocked, blamed, bound, defeated, desperate, full of dread, emotionless, exposed, horrified, in danger, inadequate, inexperienced, misunderstood, nervous, numb, out of control, overwhelmed, pressured, scattered, self-conscious, shaky, shattered, sick, spacey, stuck, threatened, vulnerable, withdrawn, young

Ambivalent: cautious, wary, confused, discombobulated, mixed, moody, needy, passive, pressured, scattered, split, torn, unclear, useless, mournful, pessimistic, regretful, remorseful, sorry, suicidal, tearful/weepy, tired, unclear, violated, worthless, wrong, numb, flat, dead

Thought Record

Situation (What were you doing or thinking about?)

_____

_____

_____

_____

Feeling(s) (1. Specify. 2. Rate 0 to 100, with 0 the lowest and 100 the highest in intensity.)

_____

_____

_____

_____

Automatic thought (What was going through your mind just before you started to feel bad? Any other thoughts?)

_____

_____

_____

_____

Facts that show it's true (List the facts.)

_____

_____

_____

_____

Facts that show it's not 100 percent true (List the facts.)

_____

_____

_____

_____

More balanced thought (What do you think now that you've looked at the facts?)

_____

_____

_____

_____

New feeling(s) (1. Specify your feelings. 2. Again, rate them on a 0 to 100 scale.)

_____

_____

_____

_____

CHAPTER 9

Mood Disorders and PMDD

The research and literature concerning PMDD have indicated that women who have a history of a depressive mood disorder or anxiety disorder may be more prone to experiencing PMDD (Bailey and Cohen 1999). As a matter of fact, PMDD can coexist with any number of mental disorders. In doctor speak, this is called *comorbidity*. It is difficult at times to isolate comorbid mood disorders because each disorder may be caused by different hormones, neurotransmitter imbalances, or life stressors. Nevertheless, it is important to identify various disorders in order to effectively treat them.

This chapter will cover the three mental disorders that most commonly coexist with PMDD—major depressive episode, dysthymia, and generalized anxiety disorder—and the complex criteria necessary to diagnose them. Several other mental disorders may also be seen together with PMDD, such as bipolar disorder, panic disorder, post-traumatic stress disorder, and seasonal affective disorder.

Mental health professionals can find the process of making an accurate diagnosis challenging at best, and frustrating at worst. The classification of mental disorders is in a constant state of refinement and development. For the most part there are no sophisticated lab and X-ray tests used in diagnosing and assessing mental disorders. Some psychologists use psychometric testing to assist them in understanding the psychological dynamics that are influencing mood and behavior. But even with psychometric testing, diagnosing a mental disorder continues to be a challenge.

You are undoubtedly aware that you have many different emotions and feelings of varying intensity going on all of the time. That's normal for everyone. You may have a day or even a week that you are tearful and sad, but that doesn't necessary mean you have a mental disorder. However, it is important to rule out the possibility of a coexisting mental disorder because effective treatment is contingent upon accurate diagnosis. This can be a very difficult and sophisticated endeavor and may require professional guidance. As you will see, the mental disorders discussed in this chapter are all very persistent, serious conditions, and not transient or monthly mood changes. They cause disruption and adverse change to major areas of your functioning at work, home, and school. Your whole world is colored by the emotions you experience in a major mental disorder. Thus, it is easy to appreciate the importance in having these disorders recognized and diagnosed correctly so appropriate treatment can begin.

Comorbidity

Comorbidity refers to the simultaneous occurrence of two of more conditions. Two important questions about comorbidity are:

1. If you meet the diagnostic criteria for both PMDD and major depressive episode or dysthymia, does that mean that one of the diagnoses are wrong?

2. Should one diagnosis be considered more important than the other?

The answer is that because PMDD and mood disorders are likely to have different causes they need to be looked at as being separate and unique.

PMDD is sometimes superimposed upon a mood disorder. In that instance of co-morbidity, it is common for the mood disorder symptoms to be exaggerated premenstrually until the PMDD subsides just after the onset of menstrual flow. This is called *premenstrual magnification*. If PMDD exists alone, all symptoms disappear within a day or two of menstrual bleeding. But if there is a comorbidity of PMDD with, let's say, a major depressive episode, the depressive symptoms abate somewhat when PMDD is over, but they don't disappear. Therefore, it is important not to dismiss premenstrual magnification of ongoing symptoms as just a fluctuation in a mood disorder, because PMDD is likely to coexist and both disorders need to be treated. Major depressive episode is frequently revealed for the first time when symptoms erroneously being attributed to PMDD fail to disappear during menstruation.

Depressive Mood Disorders

In the *DSM-IV* (APA 1994), depressive mood disorders are defined as major depressive episode and dysthymia. The severity and duration of the symptoms is what differentiates the two. Dysthymia is a long-lasting depression (over two years) in which the depressive symptoms tends to be milder.

Making the diagnosis of a mood disorder can be very difficult because it usually hinges on assessing the degree of symptom severity. What differentiates a "normal" amount of sadness from clinical depression is the degree of sadness and the impact the sadness is having on your everyday functioning in your work, school, family, and friendships, and on your effectiveness in meeting the demands of all of these different roles. Normal sadness and clinical depression display similar emotional difficulties and problems (Flett, Vredenberg, and Krames 1997). However, the person with clinical depression will have more severe and frequent symptoms that seem to last much longer (Judd et al. 1996).

Almost everyone has suffered from depression at least once in their lives. We all lose people and pets that we love. The pains and losses of growing up and growing older can cause depression. Most of the time when we experience losses, we go into a period of mourning which lightens and then eventually passes. Almost everyone will react to loss with feelings of depression—sadness, apathy, or flatness. However, a very small minority will go well beyond and develop a clinical major depressive episode or dysthymic disorder.

DSM-IV identifies four sets of symptoms in depression. They are:

- mood/feeling symptoms

- cognitive/thought symptoms

- motivational symptoms

- physical symptoms

You do not need to have symptoms in all these categories to be diagnosed as depressed, but the more symptoms that can be identified, the more accurate your diagnosis. The details follow.

DSM-IV Criteria for Major Depressive Episode

To establish the diagnosis of a major depressive episode, the following must be present:

A. Five (or more) of the following symptoms must have been present during the same two-week period and represent a change from previous functioning; at least one of the symptoms is either (1) depressed mood or (2) loss of interest or pleasure.

1. depressed mood most of the day, nearly every day, as indicated by either subjective report (e.g., feels sad or empty) or observation made by others (e.g., appears tearful)

2. markedly diminished interest or pleasure in all, or almost all, activities most of the day, nearly every day

3. significant weight loss when not dieting or weight gain (e.g., a change of more than 5 percent of body weight in a month), or decrease or increase in appetite nearly every day

4. insomnia or hypersomnia nearly every day

5. psychomotor agitation or retardation nearly every day (observable by others, not merely subjective feelings of restlessness or being slowed down)

6. fatigue or loss of energy nearly every day

7. feelings of worthlessness or excessive or inappropriate guilt nearly every day

8. diminished ability to think or concentrate, or indecisiveness, nearly every day

9. recurrent thoughts of death (not just a fear of dying), recurrent suicidal ideation without a specific plan

B. The symptoms do not meet the criteria for a mixed episode. [A mixed episode is defined as a depressive episode that is a part of a bipolar disorder. A bipolar disorder also displays a manic phase of abnormally high levels of grandiosity, a significant decrease in the need for sleep, agitated speech and motor movements, and high distractibility.]

C. The symptoms cause clinically significant distress or impairment in social, occupational, or other important areas of functioning.

D. The symptoms are not due to the direct physiological effects of a substance (e.g., a drug of abuse, a medication) or a general medical condition.

E. The symptoms are not better accounted for by bereavement, psychotic symptoms, or psychomotor retardation. (327)

As you can now appreciate, the diagnosis of major depressive episode is a rather complex undertaking.

DSM-IV *Criteria for Dysthymic Disorder*

This diagnosis is a similar exercise in information collection:

A. Depressed mood for most of the day, for more days than not, as indicated either by subjective account or observation by others, for at least two years.

B. Presence, while depressed, of two (or more) of the following:
   1. poor appetite or overeating
   2. insomnia or hypersomnia
   3. low energy or fatigue
   4. low self-esteem
   5. poor concentration or difficulty making decisions
   6. feelings of hopelessness

C. During the two-year period of the disturbance, the person has never been without the symptoms in criteria A and B for more than two months at a time.

D. No major depressive episode has been present during the first two years of the disturbance; i.e., the disturbance is not better accounted for by chronic major depressive disorder, or major depressive disorder in partial remission.

E. There has never been a manic episode.

F. The disturbance does not occur exclusively during the course of a chronic psychotic disorder.

G. The symptoms are not due to the direct physiological effects of a substance (e.g., a drug of abuse, a medication) or a general medical condition (e.g., hypothyroidism).

H. The symptoms cause clinically significant distress or impairment in social, occupational, or other important areas of functioning. (349)

Cognitive Symptoms of Depression

When you are depressed, you think of yourself, the world, and the future in a very negative manner. You may see yourself as a failure, as incompetent, inadequate, and inferior. For the most part these views of yourself, the world, and your future are distortions of reality. When depressed, you have low self-esteem and blame yourself and feel guilty for what is happening to you and around you.

Motivational Symptoms of Depression

When you are depressed, you may have trouble getting up in the morning, doing your work, getting to appointments, and making changes. In addition to the motivational problems associated with depression, many depressed people also suffer from ambivalence. You can't decide *anything*. Every decision becomes overwhelming and frightening. Fear of making the wrong decision can be paralyzing. A lack of initiative can become a "paralysis of the will."

Physical Symptoms of Depression

Depression takes the joy out of everything. Loss of appetite is common. Food loses its appeal and eating becomes too much trouble. Weight loss may occur in moderate and severe depression. In mild depression weight *gain* sometimes occurs when food becomes a comfort and a substitute, a way of avoiding and numbing the pain. Sleep disturbances are common to people with depression. You might have trouble getting to sleep at night, but more typically you suffer from what is termed early morning awakenings that leave you fatigued for the rest of the day. As a depressed person, you may also lose interest in sex and other activities that used to bring you joy and pleasure.

The following two case studies are examples of women who suffer from mood disorders and PMDD. Once diagnosed, both conditions were treated.

Major Depressive Episode and PMDD—Linda's Story

Linda is a forty-three-year-old Caucasian woman who recently lost her job at a large dot.com firm. Linda's firm is probably going to have to declare bankruptcy. She was one of the last programmers to be laid off. After losing her job, Linda cried constantly for three weeks; she reported not sleeping or eating, not wanting to spend time with family and friends, and thinking that the world would be a much better place without her. Linda said she that she lost her job because she was "an incompetent failure." She believed she might be the reason the dot.com company was going out of business. She didn't believe that she would ever be able to get another job. And she reports that she doesn't even have the energy to get out of bed and look in the want ads. The papers she needed to fill out for her unemployment insurance and COBRA benefits sat in a pile by her bed for several weeks. She just couldn't concentrate enough to fill out the paperwork.

Three years ago Linda was diagnosed with PMDD. She had been successfully working with her gynecologist and a psychologist to assist her with her PMDD symptoms. But the intensity, duration, and range of symptoms for this depression were much more severe than the depressive symptoms Linda experiences as a part of her PMDD. This observation led to Linda's diagnosis of major depressive episode.

Linda's depression could not be characterized as passing feelings of sadness and grief, but was rather an overwhelming blanket of hopelessness and helplessness. All of us occasionally have feelings of loss, sadness, and grief; these are normal responses to many of life's events. However, someone experiencing a major depressive episode feels completely overwhelmed by feelings of sadness.

Most depressions are preceded by the perception of a recent loss. In Linda's case it was the loss of her job. It can also be the breakup of a relationship, failure at work or school, rejection by a loved one, death or illness of someone close to you, and physical illness. All these are common triggers of depression (Monroe et al. 1999).

Linda's gynecologist and psychologist continued to treat her PMDD. They also began treatment for her major depressive episode. While many of the CBT techniques Linda had mastered for treating her PMDD helped in the treatment of her major depressive episode, several different and more intensive treatments were needed.

Dysthymia with PMDD—Marie's Story

Marie is a thirty-five-year-old married woman. When she was in her late twenties, both her parents were killed in an automobile accident. Marie was an only child and very close to her parents. She describes the loss of her parents as the "most traumatic event ever." She was in what she describes as a state of shock for several months after the accident. She would sit and cry for hours, wouldn't eat, and had so much trouble concentrating on anything that she needed to take an extended leave of absence from her job as a paralegal. Prior to the loss of her parents, Marie enjoyed making crafts, quilting, square dancing, and reading. She had many friends and acquaintances with whom she socialized.

Her close friends have been a strong support for Marie during this difficult time, but since losing her parents, Marie lost interest in all her prior hobbies and activities and consequently lost contact with all but a few very close friends. Although Marie returned to work, her performance suffered. She had been considered one of the best paralegals in the law office; however in the years following her loss, Marie has had problems with motivation and concentration.

After over two years of what Marie felt was "normal mourning," her husband and friends insisted that she seek out a therapist to help her come to grips with her loss. Her therapist diagnosed Marie as having dysthymia. Marie had been sad most of the day, every day for over five years. There had never been a period of longer than a couple of days that Marie did not feel this overwhelming sense of sadness and loss. She had lost interest and pleasure in activities that she used to enjoy; she suffered from fatigue, and had expressed a great deal of guilt concerning the loss of her parents. Because it had been over five years since Marie lost her parents, her situation could not be seen as a normal bereavement reaction.

In addition to the above, during the past four or five years Marie and her husband had noticed an additional pattern of depression that appears to run in conjunction with Marie's monthly menstrual cycle. They described Marie's depression becoming more severe and her becoming irritable and agitated during the week prior to the onset of her period. During that week Marie described her depressive symptoms as becoming worse, she cried more, had deeper feelings of sadness and greater hopelessness, had more trouble with insomnia and fatigue, and she had to force herself to eat. These feelings would lessen after her period started. While her depression never truly abated, the severe depressive symptoms diminished. Marie's medical doctor and her psychologist determined that Marie has both PMDD and dysthymia. She was started on antidepressant medications to help alleviate some of the symptoms, and she continued in psychotherapy to help work through the loss of her parents.

Both Marie's and Linda's cases were clear-cut examples of how PMDD can be superimposed on a major mood disorder. In both cases, PMDD resulted in premenstrual magnification of their mood disorder symptoms.

Anxiety Disorders

All of us experience feelings of fear. Fear is a normal reaction to a perceived threat or danger. There are four elements in our fear responses (Lang 1967; Rachman 1978):

1. Cognitive elements: You perceive a threat.

2. Somatic elements: Your body responds physiologically (heartbeat increases, palms get cold and sweaty, breathing gets faster and more shallow).

3. Emotional elements: You feel dread, panic, or terror.

4. Behavioral elements: You freeze, fight, or flee.

Anxiety is made up of the same four elements. The difference between anxiety and fear occurs within cognition, what you think about it. With fear you focus on a specific and clear danger. With anxiety, however, the expectation is of a more diffuse and vague danger. With fear you have a specific threatening stimulus to which you are reacting, as contrasted with anxiety, in which you are frantically searching to identify what that stimulus is, but you react nonetheless. For example, you feel fear when you are walking down a deserted street late at night and think you hear footsteps behind you. Anxiety is the feeling of being scared and full of dread when walking down a safe street filled with people in broad daylight.

DSM-IV *Criteria for Generalized Anxiety Disorder*

Generalized anxiety is chronic, and may last for months or years, with the elements of anxiety present more or less continuously. The criteria for diagnosis are:

A. Excessive anxiety and worry, occurring on more days than not for at least six months, about a number of events or activities (such as work or school performance).

B. The person finds it difficult to control the worry.

C. The anxiety and worry are associated with three (or more) of the following six symptoms (with at least some symptoms present for more days than not for the past six months).
   1. restlessness or feeling keyed up or on edge
   2. being easily fatigued
   3. difficulty concentrating or mind going blank
   4. irritability
   5. muscle tension
   6. sleep disturbance (difficulty falling or staying asleep, or restless unsatisfying sleep).

D. The focus of the anxiety and worry is not confined to features of [another] disorder.

E. The anxiety, worry, or physical symptoms cause clinically significant distress or impairment in social, occupational, or other important areas of functioning.

F. The disturbance is not due to the direct physiological effects of a substance (e.g., a drug of abuse, a medication) or a general medical condition (e.g., hyperthyroidism) and does not occur exclusively during a mood disorder, a psychotic disorder, or a pervasive developmental disorder. (435-436)

Generalized Anxiety Disorder and PMDD— Hannah's Story

Hannah is a twenty-seven-year-old German-American. She came in for psychotherapy stating that she is always uptight and worried.

From as far back as I can remember, I was scared and worried. When I was a little girl, I remember lying in my bed at night worrying that my parents or my brothers would die during the night, or that our house would catch fire or that I would strangle myself on the ribbons from my nightgown. I can remember my parents and other grown-ups telling me to smile. They'd tell me I was such a pretty little girl, but that my frown and worry lines would make me look ugly. My father was in the Army when I was little and he married my mother, who is German, while stationed in Germany. I was born in Germany, but moved to the United States when I was four. I have three younger brothers, who all never seem to have a care in the world. I was a good student and went to law school when I finished college. I just recently passed the bar exam. I should be thrilled that I have a new job as an associate in a good law firm, but I can't seem to get over my feelings that something bad is about to happen. I always have this same feeling. It's like I'm constantly waiting for the other shoe to drop, and when it drops—whoa, you'd better look out because it's gonna be nasty!

I am constantly wound up. My back and neck muscles are in knots. My boyfriend tries to give me back rubs, but he can't because I'm too tense. I have tried to give up smoking hundreds of times, but can't. Smoking seems to relax me. But after a cigarette, I picture my lungs turning black and I'm tense again waiting for a cardiac arrest! I can't relax, I pace constantly, have trouble sleeping, and never seem to laugh.

In the past couple of years I have noticed that I have become even more irritable and edgy for about a week each month. I also get really sad and blue during that same week. I started to keep track of my menstrual cycles and found that I get worse about five days before my period starts and get better right after I start my period. My doctor has prescribed some antidepressant medication and some antianxiety medication. She also recommended that I come for counseling to help me with this anxiety.

Hannah completed a diary each month which tracked her moods, anxiety levels, and menstrual cycle. It became obvious that Hannah had PMDD and had also been suffering from generalized anxiety disorder. She continued to work with her physician as well as her psychologist with cognitive behavioral techniques to help with her anxiety symptoms. She also did a lot of work in stress reduction and relaxation training. After several months, Hannah was taken off of the antianxiety medication and continued with antidepressants and cognitive behavioral therapy. Soon Hannah learned to anticipate her PMDD symptoms and to work effectively at controlling the symptoms. While still not able to completely relax, Hannah now is able to laugh, enjoy her life, and move forward in her relationship with her boyfriend. She continues on antidepressant medication and continues to work at prevention of anxiety symptoms through the cognitive behavioral techniques that she has mastered.

We included Hannah's story, and the stories of other cases of comorbidity related in this chapter, to give you some examples of how these symptoms appear in women's lives. Because of the focus of this book, it would be impossible to define and describe all of the major mental disorders and their comorbidity with PMDD. We chose to talk about major depressive episode, dysthymia, and generalized anxiety disorder because research has identified them as particularly likely to coexist with PMDD. While there is very limited research exploring comorbidity and PMDD, we assume that it can coexist with the majority of mental disorders. If you believe that you are suffering from a mental disorder plus PMDD, it is important to seek a medical and psychological consultation.

PART 4

Overview

Up to this point, our book has explained PMDD in quite some detail. You have learned what it is, how to recognize it, how to distinguish it from other disorders, and many methods for prevention and treatment. Chapter 10 will give a brief review of what we've covered, along with some suggestions for integrating this information into a useful course of action. We've also written this chapter for people important to you who may not have read the entire book, but who would benefit from a better understanding of how PMDD affects you. Finally, we've included two appendices. One offers some recipes for dishes that you will find beneficial in controlling your PMDD. The other gives you addresses and Web sites for obtaining additional information on integrative (alternative) medical therapies outlined in chapter 5.

CHAPTER 10

Tying It All Together (Plus a Word for PMDD Partners)

Premenstrual dysphoric disorder and its milder cousin, premenstrual syndrome, are conditions that women have experienced for centuries. Over all this time it has been acknowledged that these conditions exist, but until recently, the assumption was that they were simply a part of being female—something you just had to put up with because there wasn't anything to do about it. That began to change in the 1930s when adverse premenstrual symptoms were first acknowledged in medical journals. The past couple of decades have seen a quantum leap forward. We have seen:

- grudging recognition by skeptics that PMDD and PMS are real

- research discoveries that PMDD/PMS have biological origins

- a reliable means to diagnose these conditions and distinguish them from each other, as well as from mental disorders

- effective treatment regimens to address physical as well as psychological symptoms

This chapter will briefly summarize the management interventions available to you if you suffer from PMDD. We also have addressed a section of this chapter to your partner. Urge your partner, or anyone else important to your everyday life, to read it. People close to you will benefit from a thumbnail sketch of PMDD/PMS. If they know that what happens to you on a regular monthly basis is not of your doing or in your immediate control, their understanding will help you in your effort to control your PMDD.

After Diagnosis, Then What?

You should review your two-month daily symptom-rating diary (see chapter 2). This will demonstrate graphically to you whether or not your premenstrual symptoms and their pattern of appearance and disappearance are consistent with PMDD. Find out the results of any diagnostic tests for other conditions (e.g., hypothyroidism, diabetes, anemia, systemic lupus, mood disorders). Knowing the results of your diagnostic workup will help remove doubt from your mind as to what is happening to you. Just knowing the type, severity, and timing of your premenstrual symptoms can make them seem more manageable.

Treatment of Any Coexisting Physical or Psychiatric Conditions

Treatment of any physical condition (e.g., hypothyroidism) or psychiatric disorder (e.g., depression) should be first on your doctor's management agenda. By eliminating the symptoms of such conditions, you may find your premenstrual symptoms will disappear or be significantly diminished.

If other medical illnesses have been ruled out, you can then see which of five diagnostic categories apply to you:

1. You have PMS.

2. You have PMDD.

3. You have PMDD or PMS coexisting with a psychiatric disorder.

4. You have only a psychiatric disorder and no PMDD or PMS.

5. You have neither PMDD/PMS nor a psychiatric disorder.

With your diagnostic category established, the obvious next step is to select the appropriate interventions.

Management Options

You have a number of different options. First let's look at how you might go about treating the most troubling symptoms.

Self-Help

The self-help measures covered in chapters 3, 4, and 5 are good places to start. These are the means for you to alter your lifestyle so as to not only help your PMDD/PMS symptoms directly but also to establish a sense of wellness in your life. If you can achieve the type of wellness described in the opening paragraph of chapter 3, your PMDD/PMS will be very favorably modified. This involves good nutrition, weight control, adequate exercise, elimination of destructive habits (smoking, alcohol, and substance abuse), informed use of vitamin and mineral supplements, and perhaps the employment of integrative (alternative) medical therapies. As explained in chapter 5, this latter form of treatment for PMDD/PMS is not yet well-grounded in reliable science. Nevertheless, botanical therapy and other disciplines, such as homeopathy, naturopathy, traditional Chinese medicine, Ayurvedic medicine, and craniosacral therapy, help many women who suffer from PMDD/PMS.

Medication Help

If your diagnosis is PMDD, disruptive mood symptoms are the most prominent aspect of your premenstrual symptoms. That's a given. If they are of sufficient magnitude to interfere with your everyday functioning in the family, social, and vocational spheres of your life, then you are a candidate for pharmacological treatment. In your situation, this may be the most appropriate initial therapy for you. Fortunately, effective drug therapy is available in the form of selective serotonin reuptake inhibitors, discussed in chapter 6. Other psychotropic drugs are also available, but none has the track record of the SSRIs. If your doctor suggests SSRI treatment, give it the serious consideration that credible research has shown it deserves.

Emotional Help

Chapter 7 addressed how you can reduce your PMDD if you take steps to control stress in your life. PMDD sufferers are now known to have an abnormal biological response to stress. We don't yet have a means of favorably altering your abnormal stress response, but much is known about how you can more favorably deal with stress itself. It's easy to learn these techniques, so take advantage of them.

Chapter 8 explained a newer method of PMDD management called cognitive behavioral therapy (CBT). CBT has been in use for mood disorders (e.g., depression) for several decades, but its value in treating PMDD has only recently been demonstrated. CBT teaches you to evaluate and alter your negative thinking patterns, the hallmark of PMDD, so that you can successfully deal with those horrendous moods that possess you on a monthly basis. You'll need a psychologist to teach you CBT techniques, but once you learn how to use CBT, you can manage nicely on your own.

Menstrual Cycle Manipulation As Treatment

You know from chapter 6 that PMDD/PMS only occurs if you are having normal menstrual cycles. If you do not ovulate, you don't have PMDD/PMS. This information has led to five methods for controlling premenstrual symptoms based on altering the hormonal milieu of your cycle, or by stopping ovulation.

1. **Estrogen if you are premenopausal.** If you are in your forties and experiencing PMDD for the first time, an estrogen supplement can stop your PMDD symptoms.

2. **Oral contraceptives (OCs).** OCs suppress ovulation and hormone production by your ovaries, so PMDD symptoms are controlled. A new OC called Yasmin is demonstrating better than average results in controlling PMDD symptoms. Ask your doctor about it.

3. **GnRH agonists.** These hormones control PMDD effectively by stopping ovarian function. They also create a false menopause with all the accompanying estrogen-depletion symptoms such as hot flashes, moodiness, vaginal dryness, and short-term memory deficits.

4. **Danocrine.** This is a male hormone derivative that stops pituitary stimulation of your ovaries and shuts them down. It works, but the side effects are usually unacceptable for most women.

5. **Ovariectomy.** Surgical removal of both ovaries is quite effective in stopping PMDD, but it results in instant menopause with all the accompanying estrogen-deficient symptoms. Estrogen replacement therapy can help, but not completely enough for young women.

On the Horizon

Since PMDD is acknowledged to be the result of an abnormal neurotransmitter response to normal female hormone production, research is homing in on how best to use this information. The current view of researchers is that low levels of circulating serotonin constitute the major abnormality that results in PMDD. Several selective serotonin reuptake inhibitors (SSRIs) have been shown to be useful in preventing low serotonin levels.

In spite of this, up to 40 percent of PMDD sufferers are not helped by SSRIs. This is thought to be because currently available SSRIs are not specific enough in attaching to the appropriate brain cell receptor site.

Six serotonin receptor types are known to exist. As understanding of each of their functions improves, a new generation of SSRIs will be developed that will be able to attach to only those receptor sites that influence PMDD or depressive symptoms. Citalopram, marketed under the trade name Celexa, is a model for this kind of new drug. It has the same usefulness as other SSRIs in treating PMDD symptoms, but without the sexual side effects associated with these drugs.

Continuing studies of other neurotransmitters (norepinephrine, GABA, allopregnanolone) are underway to find yet additional methods and medications to control PMDD. So, the future looks bright.

Just for PMDD Partners

If your partner suffers from premenstrual dysphoric disorder, you have an important role to play in helping her control her monthly turmoil. It is hoped this section can also be useful for family members, friends (even enemies), coworkers, and others with whom she regularly comes in contact.

You are probably aware that the symptoms of PMDD/PMS are commonly treated as jokes in sitcoms, movies, and in real life to account for aggressive female behavior. For your partner, however, it's anything but funny. During her PMDD days, she knows her attitudes and behaviors are often not appropriate. She knows that she's not at her best during these times, and it can be very frustrating for her. She often does not feel in control.

What You Can Do

Perhaps the most important thing you can do for your partner is to convey to her that you are *there* for her. She needs to know that you understand what PMDD is, and what it does to her. If you know something about this disorder, and recognize when she is in the grip of her monthly chaos, your knowledge can help her. You can't solve the problems confronting your partner, but if you are supportive and even-tempered, her chances of coping with them well are greatly improved.

Reassure her that you find her attractive. Many women have very low self-esteem during their PMDD days, and you can help to support her. Warm, honest hugs (lots of them) say volumes about how you feel about her.

Listen to her attentively as she mulls over the options available for controlling her PMDD. Your opinion might even be solicited if she feels you have done your homework and learned some useful information about the monthly turmoil that besets her. Positive support and feedback from you will make it easier for her to decide from among the various options for self-help and/or third party help that are available.

As already discussed, PMDD is a subset of PMS characterized by severe mood derangements. You can't prevent her ferocious mood upheavals, but you can avoid aggravating them. When you recognize her PMDD is occurring, don't bring up divisive issues that can trigger her anger and rage. Write down the problem you wish to discuss, and try to defer the discussion for calmer times. This doesn't mean that you must swallow your words for fear of her wrath every time you have concerns. You have needs and rights also. It just makes it more probable that you will have a productive discussion if she is not suffering from PMDD.

If your partner *is* shooting rats with cannons because you forgot to pick up the dry cleaning on your way home, Dr. Lonnie Barbach, a psychologist at the University of California in San Francisco, suggests that you regard the intensity of her reaction as only about one-tenth of what it seems (Barbach 1993). Then admit to the underlying validity of her complaint (you *did* forget that damn dry cleaning) and withdraw from the field of battle. Nothing productive is accomplished by your angrily pointing out her exaggerated response to your minor error. Later, when she has regained her composure, she will appreciate your understanding.

From the preceding discussion in this chapter, we hope you can conclude that premenstrual dysphoric disorder is a complex condition for which we don't have all the answers. Nevertheless, intense research in the past thirty years has produced some very useful information, which is helping us better understand and treat PMDD. As a PMDD partner, you have immense power to make an enormous difference for a woman who is suffering this cyclic turmoil. Through understanding and support, you can be of unlimited help in her taking control of her PMDD. Some friction and conflict is inevitable of course; but if the two of you can deal with it successfully, it will initiate new growth in your relationship.

Billing for PMDD

When you see your doctor for PMDD, be sure the charges are billed correctly. Every medical diagnosis has an assigned number from the ICD-9-CM code. At present, PMDD does not have an assigned ICD-9-CM code number that is different from PMS. The code that comes closest to characterizing PMS or PMDD is 625.4 for "premenstrual tension syndromes." This code doesn't capture some of the mood derangement aspects of PMDD, but it represents a recognized condition that will not normally be challenged for payment by insurance companies.

Some billing clerks try to be more specific and accurate in billing for PMDD. In addition to the 625.4 coding for PMS, they may add codes for depression, anxiety, or emotional liability: "depressive disorder, not else-where classified" (311); "anxiety state, unspecified" (300); "affective personality disorder, unspecified" (301.1); "explosive personality disorder" (301.3). The problem with these codes is that they are in the mental disorders chapter of the ICD-9-CM code book. Using them may lead to future insurance payment problems for you because they label you as mentally ill. This can create problems for you if:

1. You do not have mental health coverage.

2. Your insurance recognizes only a psychiatrist or psychologist as a qualified provider for these diagnoses.

3. You have limited coverage for mental health, and using these codes results in a higher copayment or a time limit on treatment.

One of our major goals for this book has been to present a rather complex topic in an understandable way. If you've gotten to this point, then perhaps we have succeeded. We presented a number of techniques and treatment methods for coping with PMDD in order to better empower you to take control of this chaotic monthly incursion in your life.

Our wish for you as our reader is that you will be successful in making the lifestyle changes that can help your PMDD. If they do not help enough, you must not hesitate to seek pharmacological treatment or psychological care. You now know that both can help you.

Finally, we urge you to diligently pursue achieving control of your PMDD. It is too life-altering to do otherwise. Our belief is that this isn't a dress rehearsal you are going through. It is your life and we hope the information in this book will help you to control your PMDD so you can make it the best life possible.

Appendix A

Sample Recipes

You can reduce your PMDD symptoms by improving your diet. Simply eat more complex carbohydrates and less animal protein during the ten days prior to your menstrual period. The recipes that follow are designed to follow this principle and still be nutritious, tasty, and convenient.

Foods to emphasize

- **seafood:** shrimp, crab, oysters, tuna, salmon
- **poultry:** skinless turkey or chicken, broiled or baked
- **vegetables:** tomatoes, peppers, potatoes, all green vegetables
- **fruits:** strawberries, blackberries, oranges, apricots, cantaloupe, watermelon
- **whole grain foods:** barley and oat products, pita bread
- **pasta:** whole wheat is good, several specialty pastas too
- **rice:** brown rice
- **legumes:** lentis and beans; good additives for salads, meat-free chili, soups, and dips
- **nuts:** almonds, walnuts, sunflower seeds

Foods to minimize

- **red meat:** cured, smoked, or processed beef, bacon, and sausages
- **dairy products:** milk, cheese, cream, ice cream
- **sugars:** jams, maple syrup, dried fruits

- **sweets:** candy, cake, cookies, pastry
- **snack foods:** potato chips, corn chips, snack crackers, nachos
- **fast foods, convenience foods:** most are loaded with salt
- **coffee, tea, colas:** too much caffeine
- **white flour products:** no nutritional value

Grilled Chicken with Pasta and Spinach

Plenty of potassium, carotene, vitamin cup, and folic acid (B_9). Also a good source of complex carbohydrates, vitamin E, and vitamin B_6.

3 cups penne pasta

2 to 3 teaspoons olive oil

2 chicken breasts, boned and skinned, sliced into ½-inch strips

1 small red onion, cut in ½-inch wedges

3 cloves garlic or to taste

½ pound mushrooms, sliced

1 large red pepper, thinly sliced

1 large yellow or orange pepper, thinly sliced

½ cup dry white wine or vermouth

1 bag baby spinach

Zest and juice of ½ lemon

1 tablespoon chopped fresh parsley

1 tablespoon chopped fresh basil

Black pepper to taste

Cook the pasta according to package directions and set aside. Heat 2 teaspoons olive oil in a wok. Add the chicken and stir-fry for 1½ minutes, then remove from the wok. Add the onions and garlic to the wok. Sauté for 2 to 3 minutes making sure the garlic doesn't burn. You may need to add another teaspoon of olive oil for cooking the vegetables. To the onion mixture, add mushrooms, red and yellow peppers and stir-fry 1 minute. Now pour the white wine into the wok, boiling for 3 minutes until liquid is partially reduced. Add spinach and cover wok for 1 minute of steaming. Return the already cooked chicken and pasta to the wok and stir to blend all ingredients. Add the lemon juice and zest, parsley, basil, and black pepper to taste.

Warm plates or serving bowls in advance to keep pasta hot. Parmesan cheese sounds tempting, but you probably should pass on it. Serves 4 as a main course.

Shrimp (or Chicken Breast) Stir-fry

Fast, delicious, and healthy.

2 teaspoons olive oil

12 jumbo shrimp (could substitute 1 chicken breast, skinned and cut into strips)

2 cloves garlic, chopped

2 teaspoons fresh ginger, peeled and chopped. (Okay to use more if you like ginger)

1 red bell pepper, thinly sliced

12 to 15 snow pea pods

4 green onions, cut into 2-inch pieces

Heat the oil in a wok or skillet. Add the shrimp, garlic, and ginger and sauté for 2 minutes (if using chicken, sauté 3 to 4 minutes). Add the peppers and pea pods, stirring for 1 minute. Add the green onions last and stir 1 minute. Serve on a bed of brown or jasmine rice. Serves two.

Grilled Halibut with Citrus Salsa

Features plenty of vitamins, minerals, and omega-3 fatty acid all of which help with PMDD/PMS. A great BBQ accompanied with steamed asparagus and brown rice.

6 1-inch halibut steaks, each 6 ounces

Pesto for BBQ sauce:
2 tablespoons fresh lemon juice

1 teaspoon olive oil

2 tablespoons pine nuts

1 bunch fresh basil

Citrus salsa:
2 tablespoons fresh cilantro

¼ cup red onion

1 red grapefruit

1 navel orange

1 jalapeno pepper

1 tablespoon honey

Combine all pesto ingredients and puree. Spread the pesto sauce on halibut and turn pesto side down on grill on medium heat for 5 minutes. Spread the pesto sauce on the uncooked side and flip over, grilling another 5 minutes. Serve with citrus salsa topping.

For salsa, peel grapefruit and orange. Combine all ingredients in food chopper until chunky. Serves 6.

Citrus-Roasted Salmon

This recipe with a citrus touch is ideal for company.

1 teaspoon grated lemon

2 tablespoons fresh lemon juice

2 tablespoons honey

4 teaspoons chili powder

1 teaspoon ground cumin

½ teaspoon salt

½ teaspoon ground coriander seeds

¼ teaspoon ground red pepper

1 (6 ounces) can thawed orange juice concentrate

4 (6 ounces) salmon fillets, skinned, 1 inch thick

Cooking spray

Orange wedges (optional)

Flat-leaf parsley sprigs (optional)

Combine lemon, lemon juice, honey, chili powder, cumin, salt, coriander seeds, red pepper, and orange juice in a bowl. Brush both sides of fish with this juice mixture. Save remaining juice. Place the fish fillets on a broiler pan coated with cooking spray. Preheat the oven to 400° F and bake for 15 minutes or until the fish flakes easily when tested with a fork.

Place leftover orange juice mixture in a small sauce pan, bring to a boil, and cook until reduced to ½ cup (about 2 minutes). Serve 2 tablespoons with each fish fillet and garnish with orange wedges and parsley. Serves 4.

Grilled Chicken Breasts with Plum Salsa

An interesting twist to chicken!

Chicken:

2 teaspoons brown sugar

½ teaspoon salt

½ teaspoon ground cumin

¼ teaspoon garlic powder

4 (4 ounces) chicken breast halves, skinned, boneless

2 teaspoons vegetable oil

Plum Salsa:

1 cup chopped ripe plum (about 2 plums)
(Peaches, nectarines, or pineapple can be substituted for plums)

2 tablespoons chopped fresh cilantro or 1 teaspoon dried

2 tablespoons red onion, chopped

2 teaspoons cider vinegar

¼ teaspoon hot sauce

⅛ teaspoon salt

Combine the brown sugar, salt, cumin, and garlic powder, and rub on the chicken breasts. Heat the oil in a non-stick skillet over medium heat. Add the chicken; cook 6 minutes on each side. While the chicken is cooking, combine the salsa ingredients in a bowl. Serve ¼ cup salsa with each chicken breast. Serves 4.

Fresh Vegetable Salad

A light and refreshing salad.

2 cups snow peas

1 cup sliced zucchini, one yellow, one green

1 cup carrots, thinly sliced

1 red or yellow pepper, thinly sliced

1 cup cooked fresh corn (frozen okay, but fresh much better)

¼ cup olive oil

2 tablespoons fresh peppermint leaves, chopped (or 1 teaspoon dried)

2 tablespoons fresh lime or lemon juice

Grated rind from 1 small lemon (optional)

Black pepper to taste

Blanch the snow peas, zucchini, and carrots for 2 minutes. Drain well. Place in a serving bowl. Add the red pepper and fresh corn. Drizzle with oil, adding mint, lemon juice, lemon rind, and pepper. Toss and marinate at least 1 hour. Bring to room temperature. Toss again before serving. Serves 6 to 8.

Autumn Acorn Squash Soup

As the leaves are changing and the evenings take on a brisk nip, soup is a natural meal. This is a good soup for lunch or a first course for dinner.

2 medium acorn squashes, peeled, seeded, and cubed

2 tablespoons olive oil

1 large onion, chopped

1 cup carrots, coarsely chopped

¾ teaspoon nutmeg

1 tablespoon brown sugar

1 teaspoon grated ginger

½ teaspoon cinnamon

3 cans salt-free chicken broth

Rosemary sprig garnish (optional)

Place the squash pieces in 1 inch of water and cook for 15 minutes. Remove the pulp. Add the olive oil, onion, carrots, nutmeg, sugar, ginger, and cinnamon. Cover the pot and simmer for 15 minutes. Add 3 cups of chicken broth and puree in a blender. Add the remaining chicken broth, bring to a boil, and add a rosemary sprig (if desired). Cook for 10 minutes more. Serves 4 to 6.

Tabbouleh Wheat Salad

A taste treat from an ancient Middle Eastern recipe.

1 package tabbouleh wheat salad mix (located with packaged rices or in the gourmet section of your market)

1 cup fresh tomatoes, chopped

1 tablespoon fresh lemon juice, 2 tablespoons if you like a more tart flavor

1 tablespoon olive oil

½ cup red pepper, chopped

¼ cup fresh basil, chopped

½ cup green onions, chopped

In a large bowl, combine the wheat salad mix and the contents of the accompanying spice pack. Stir in 1 cup boiling water. Cover and let stand 30 minutes in the refrigerator. Add the above ingredients. Refrigerate 4 hours or overnight to let flavors blend. Serve on a bed of lettuce. Serves 6 to 8.

Optional condiments:
Black olives, mint, cayenne pepper, cucumbers

For a fruit tabbouleh wheat salad, add 1 cup blueberries or mandarin oranges

Walnut and Pasta Salad

A tangy and nutritious salad.

8 ounces medium pasta shells, uncooked

1½ cups red grapes

1 cup celery

2 oranges, medium, navel, peeled and sliced

1 apple, peeled, cored, coarsely chopped

½ cup walnuts

Dressing:

1 tablespoon honey

¼ cup frozen orange juice concentrate, thawed

1 cup non-fat plain yogurt

Prepare the pasta according to the directions on the package and drain. Mix the honey, orange juice, and yogurt together in a bowl. Add the pasta, grapes, orange slices and celery to the yogurt mixture. Toss, cover, and chill overnight. Just before serving, add the apple and nuts. Serve 6 to 8 for lunch or a light dinner main course.

Basic Vinaigrette

Many commercial salad dressings contain as much as 330 milligrams of sodium per tablespoon. If you suffer from PMDD, you can appreciate that too much salt contributes to breast tenderness, bloating, and fluid retention. Instead of using the prepared stuff, why not make your own?

5 tablespoons olive oil

2 tablespoons balsamic vinegar

1 teaspoon dried tarragon leaves

Mix well. Serve over salad greens or steamed veggies. Makes about ½ cup.

Italian Style Dressing and Marinade

You can make your own with less fat than commercial brands. This has no cholesterol, is low in saturated fat, and emphasizes monounsaturated fat.

¼ cup red wine vinegar

⅔ cup olive oil

2 to 3 cloves garlic, minced, or chopped

1 tablespoon fresh lemon juice

1 sprig fresh rosemary or 1 teaspoon dried

2 teaspoons fresh oregano or 1 teaspoon dried

¼ teaspoon coarsely ground black pepper

Process all ingredients in blender for 2 minutes. Refrigerate in an airtight glass container. Makes 1 cup.

Can be sprinkled over fresh greens, pasta, brussels sprouts, green beans, or a vegetable of your preference. Excellent for marinating fish or chicken breasts.

Roasted Potatoes

This potato preparation can accompany any main course.

4 peeled and quartered potatoes (can also use small red potatoes, skins on)

2 tablespoons olive oil

2 tablespoons lemon juice

1 teaspoon dried oregano

½ teaspoon dried rosemary, 1 teaspoon if fresh

2 garlic cloves, minced

Black pepper to taste

In a bowl, combine all the ingredients except the potatoes. Stir well, then coat the potatoes with the oil mixture. Stir well, coat the potatoes with the oil mixture. Place the potatoes on a lightly greased baking pan. Bake at 425° F for 1 hour. Stir every 15 minutes until cooked and crisp.

Oat Bran Muffins

This recipe is a healthy alternative to cookies and other pastries. It is also an excellent breakfast food. Sunflower seeds are a good source of vitamin E and linoleic acid (a component of omega-3 fatty acid, the PMDD fighter).

1½ cups oat bran

2 teaspoons ground cinnamon

2 teaspoons baking powder

1 large apple

1 inch strip lemon rind

3 tablespoons water

¾ cup skim milk

1 egg white

¼ cup dark raisins

¼ cup sunflower seeds, raw, shelled, unsalted

Olive oil for muffin tins

Combine the oat bran, cinnamon, and baking powder in a bowl. Puree the apple, lemon rind, water, milk, and egg white, then stir into the oat bran mixture with the raisins and sunflower seeds. Wait 10 to 15 minutes for the mixture to thicken. Preheat oven to 400° F. Brush muffin tins with oil, add batter, and bake for 15 to 18 minutes until muffins begin to brown. They last for about 4 days, but you can make a large batch and freeze them for future consumption.

Breakfast Pumpkin Muffins

Pumpkin is a healthy food, loaded with complex carbohydrates, fiber, and potassium.

1 cup fresh cooked pumpkin

½ cup water

2 tablespoons honey

½ cup canola oil

2 cups unsifted flour

½ cup packed dark brown sugar

1 teaspoon baking soda

½ teaspoon cinnamon

½ teaspoon ginger

⅛ teaspoon nutmeg

⅓ cup coarsely chopped walnuts

To cook the pumpkin, peel and cut it into 1 inch cubes. Boil them in a small amount of water until tender. Process in a blender until thick and smooth. Combine the pumpkin with water, honey, and canola oil, and stir.

In a large bowl, combine the flour, brown sugar, baking soda, cinnamon, ginger, and nutmeg. Add the pumpkin mixture to dry ingredients, and stir. Add walnuts, and spoon into greased muffin tins. Bake at 375° F for 20 minutes. Makes 12 muffins.

Fresh Fruit Drink

Loaded with vitamins. Good for breakfast or snacks.

   1 cup orange juice, fresh or from concentrate

   10 strawberries

   2 bananas

Combine the ingredients in a blender with 6 ice cubes for about 30 seconds. The unused portion can be refrigerated. Makes 3 cups.

Watermelon Drink

Watermelon is a good source for potassium, which is known to be helpful in controlling premenstrual bloating, fatigue, and irritability.

   1½ cups watermelon, seedless, diced

   1 tablespoon fresh lemon juice

   ¾ cup lemon sorbet

Blend with 6 ice cubes until smooth. Makes 3 cups.

APPENDIX B

Resources for Integrative Medical Therapies

For a government compendium about food supplements discussed in chapter 5, go to www.nal.usda.gov/fnic/IBIDS. Go to http://vm. cfsan.fds.gov/_dms/supplmnt.html for additional information about dietary supplements and herbal interactions with other drugs. For information on alternative medical disciplines discussed in chapter 5, contact the following organizations.

American Association of Acupuncture and Oriental Medicine: 433 Front Street, Catasaqua, PA 18032; (610) 433-2448; http://www.aaom. org

American Association of Naturopathic Physicians: www.naturopathic.org or www.aanp.org

National Center for Homeopathy: 810 North Fairfax Street, Suite 306, Alexandria, VA 22314; (704) 548-7790; www.homeopathic.org

National Institute of Ayurvedic Medicine: 584 Milltown Road, Brewster, NY 10509; (845) 278-8700; www.niam.com

The Upledger Institute for Complementary Care and Education: 11211 Prosperity Farms Road, Suite D-325, Palm Beach Gardens, FL 34410; (800) 233-5880; www.upledger.com for information on craniosacral therapy

References

Chapter 1
What Is PMDD and Who Gets It?

ACOG (American College of Obstetricians and Gynecologists). 2000. Premenstrual syndrome: clinical management guidelines for obstetrician-gynecologists. *ACOG Practice Bulletin* 15:1-9.

APA (American Psychiatric Association). 1994. *Diagnostic and Statistical Manual of Mental Disorders*. 4th ed. Washington, D.C.: APA.

Frye, G. M., and S. D. Silverman. 2000. Is it premenstrual syndrome? Keys to focused diagnosis, therapies for multiple symptoms. *Postgraduate Medicine* 107:151-159.

Kaplan, A. G. 1986. The "self in relation": Implications for depression in women. *Psychotherapy: Theory, Research, and Practice* 23:235–242

Mortola, J. F. 1994. A risk-benefit appraisal of drugs used in the management of premenstrual syndrome. *Drug Safety* 10:260-169.

Parker, P. D. 1994. Premenstrual syndrome. *American Family Physician* 50:1309-1317.

Pearlstein, T. B., and A. B. Stone. 1998. Premenstrual syndrome. *Psychiatric Clinics of North America* 21:577-590.

Steiner, M., and A. Wilkins. 1996. Diagnosis and assessment of premenstrual dysphoria. *Psychiatric Annals* 26(9):571-575.

Women's Health Research. 1999. www.information@womens-health.org (5/28/01).

Woods, N. F., et al. 1986. *Prevalence of Premenstrual Symptoms*. Washington, D.C.: U.S. Public Health Service, Division of Nursing; Final Report NLL 1054.

World Health Organization. 1996. *International Classification of Diseases*. 10th rev. Geneva, Switzerland: World Health Organization.

Chapter 2
Medical Information: What's Known, What Isn't

ACOG (American College of Obstetricians and Gynecologists), 2000. Premenstrual Syndrome: Clinical Management Guidelines for Obstetrician-Gynecologists. *ACOG Practice Bulletin* 15:1-9.

APA (American Psychiatric Association). 1994. *Diagnostic and Statistical Manual of Mental Disorders.* 4th ed. Washington, D.C.: APA.

Bailey, J. W., and L. S. Cohen. 1999. Prevalence of mood and anxiety disorders in women who seek treatment for premenstrual syndrome. *Journal of Women's Health and Gender Based Medicine* 8(9):1181-1184.

British Columbia Reproductive Mental Health Program. 2001. www.bcrmh.com/disorders/pms.htm (5/28/01).

Condon, J. T. 1993. The premenstrual syndrome: A twin study. *British Journal of Psychiatry* 162:481-486.

Eriksson, E. 1999. Serotonin reuptake inhibitors for the treatment of premenstrual dysphoric disorder. *International Clinics in Psychopharmacology* 14(suppl. 2): S25-31.

Girdler, S. S. 2000. Women with PMDD are more sensitive to pain. Paper presented at the annual meeting of the *American Psychosomatic Society,* in Atlanta.

Girdler, S. S., et al. 1998. Dysregulation of cardiovascular and neuroendocrine responses to stress in premenstrual dysphoric disorder. *Psychiatry Research* 81(2):163-178.

Girdler, S. S., et al. 2001. Allopregnanolone levels and reactivity to mental illness in premenstrual dysphoric disorder. *Biological Psychiatry* 49(9):788-797.

Huston, J. E., and L. D. Lanka. 2001. *Perimenopause: Changes in Women's Health After 35.* Oakland, Calif.: New Harbinger Publications.

Kaleli, S., et al. 2001. Lisuride maleate provides symptomatic relief of premenstrual breast pain. *Fertility and Sterility* 75:718-723.

Kessel, S. 2000. Premenstrual syndrome: Advances in diagnosis and treatment. *Obstetrical and Gynecological Clinics of North America* 27(3):625-639

Mortola J. F. 1992. Issues in the diagnosis and research of premenstrual syndrome. *Clinical Obstetrics and Gynecology* 35:587-598.

———. 1995. Pathophysiology and treatment of premenstrual syndrome. *Current Opinion in Endocrinology and Diabetes* 2:483-490.

———. 1997. From GnRH to SSRIs and Beyond: Weighing the Options for Drug Therapy in Premenstrual Syndrome. *Medscape Women's Health* 2(10); www.medscape.com (8/1/01).

Mortola, J. F., et al. 1990. Diagnosis of premenstrual syndrome by a simple, prospective, and reliable instrument: the calendar of premenstrual experiences. *Obstetrics and Gynecology* 76:302-307.

Pearlstein, T. B., and A. B. Stone. 1998. Premenstrual syndrome. *Psychiatric Clinics of North America* 21:577-590.

Praschak-Rieder, N., et al. 2001. Prevalence of premenstrual dysphoric disorder in female patients with seasonal affective disorder. *Journal of Affective Disorders* 63(1-3):239-242.

Reid, R. L. 1985. Premenstrual syndrome. *Current Problems in Obstetrics, Gynecology, and Fertility* 8:1-57.

Schmidt, P. J., L. K. Nieman, and M. A. Danaceau. 1998. Differential behavioral effects of gonadal steroids in women with and in those without premenstrual syndrome. *New England Journal of Medicine* 338:209-216.

Steiner, M. 2000. Premenstrual syndrome and premenstrual dysphoric disorder: Guidelines for management. *Journal of Psychiatry & Neuroscience* 25(5):459-468.

Steiner, M., S. Steinberg, and D. Stewart. 1995. Fluoxetine in the treatment of premenstrual dysphoria. *New England Journal of Medicine* 332:1529-1534.

Steiner, M., and A. Wilkins. 1996. Diagnosis and assessment of premenstrual dysphoria. *Psychiatric Annals* 26(9):571-575.

Thys-Jacobs, S., et al. 1998. Calcium carbonate and the premenstrual syndrome: Effects on premenstrual and menstrual symptoms. *American Journal of Obstetrics and Gynecology* 178(2):444-452.

World Health Organization. 1987. *Mental, Behavioral and Developmental Disorders.* 10th revision of the International Classification of Diseases (1986 draft for field trials). Geneva, Switzerland: World Health Organization.

Yonkers, K. A. 1997. The association between premenstrual dysphoric disorder and other mood disorders. *Journal of Clinical Psychiatry* 58(suppl. 15):S19-25.

———. 1999. Medical management of premenstrual dysphoric disorder. *Journal of Gender-Specific Medicine* 2(3):55-60.

Chapter 3
Nutritional Help for PMDD

Albert, C. M., et al. 1998. Fish consumption and the risk of sudden cardiac death. *Journal of the American Medical Association* 279(1):23-28.

Bellerson, K. 1993. *The Complete Fat Book.* Garden City Park, N.Y.: Avery Publishing.

Bendich, A. 2000. The potential for dietary supplements to reduce premenstrual syndrome (PMS) symptoms. *Journal of the American College of Nutritionists* 19:3-12.

Bland, J. S. 1999. *Genetic Nutritioneering.* Los Angeles: Keats Publishing.

Caan, B., D. Duncan, and R. Hiatt. 1993. Association between alcoholic and caffeinated beverages and premenstrual syndrome. *Journal of Reproductive Medicine* 38:630-636

Cutler, W., and C. R. Garcia. 1992. *Menopause: A Guide for Women and the Men Who Love Them.* New York: W.W. Norton.

Daoust, J., and G. Daoust. 1996. *Fat Burning Nutrition.* Del Mar, Calif.: Wharton Publishing.

Daugherty, J. E. 1998. Treatment strategies for premenstrual syndrome. *American Family Physician* 58:183-192, 197-198.

Facchinetti, F., et al. 1991. Oral magnesium successfully relieves premenstrual mood changes. *Obstetrics and Gynecology* 78:177.

Harvard Heart Letter. 2000. Women and heart disease. *Harvard Heart Letter* 10(5):1-4.

Hu, F. B. 1999. A prospective study of egg consumption and risk of cardiovascular disease in men and women. *Journal of the American Medical Association* 281:1384-1394.

Huston, J. E., and L. D. Lanka. 2001. *Perimenopause: Changes in Women's Health After 35.* Oakland, Calif.: New Harbinger Publications.

Institute of Medicine. 1997. *Dietary References Intakes: Calcium, Phosphorus, Magnesium, Vitamin D, and Fluoride.* Washington, D.C.: National Academy Press.

Johns Hopkins Health Letter. 2001. Reevaluating your cholesterol. *Johns Hopkins Medical Letter: Health After 50* 13(6):1-2.

Kromhaut, D., E. Bosschieter, and C. Coulander. 1985. The inverse relation between fish consumption and 20 year mortality from coronary heart disease. *New England Journal of Medicine* 312:1205-1209.

Lapidus, L. 1986. Ischemic heart disease, stroke, and mortality in women: Results from a prospective population study in Gothenburg, Sweden. *Acta Medicus Scandinavia* (suppl.) 219:1-42.

McDowell, M. A., et al. 1994. *Third National Health and Nutrition Examination Survey with Data from National Center for Health Statistics.* Washington, D.C.: Government Printing Office.

Ojeda, L. 1995. *Menopause without Medicine.* Alameda, Calif.: Hunter House.

Parker, P. D. 1994. Premenstrual syndrome. *American Family Physician* 50:1309-1317.

Penland, J. G., and P. E. Johnson. 1993. Dietary calcium and manganese effects on menstrual cycle symptoms. *American Journal of Obstetrics and Gynecology* 168:1417-1423.

Rossignol, A. M., and H. Bonnlander. 1991. Prevalence and severity of the premenstrual syndrome. Effects of foods and beverages that are sweet or high in sugar content. *Journal of Reproductive Medicine* 36:131-136.

Severino, S. K., and M. L. Moline. 1995. Premenstrual syndrome. Identification and management. *Drugs. Practical Therapeutics* 49(1):71–82.

Steinberg, S. L., et al. 1999. A placebo-controlled clinical trail of L-tryptophan in premenstrual dysphoria. *Biological Psychiatry* 45(3):313-320.

Takacs, B. E. 1998. Potassium: A new treatment for premenstrual syndrome. *Journal of Orthomolecular Medicine* 13:215-222.

Thys-Jacobs, S., et al. 1998. Calcium carbonate and the premenstrual syndrome: effects on premenstrual and menstrual symptoms. *American Journal of Obstetrics and Gynecology* 178(2):444-452.

Walker, A. F., M. C. DeSouza, and M. F. Vickers. 1998. Magnesium supplementation alleviates premenstrual symptoms of fluid retention. *Journal of Women's Health* 7:1157-1165.

Willet, W. 1994. Diet and health: What should we eat? *Science* 264:532-537.

Willet, W., M. Stampfer, and J. Manson. 1993. Intake of trans fatty acids and risks of coronary heart disease among women. *Lancet* 341:581-585.

Wyatt, K. M., et al. 1999. Efficacy of vitamin B-6 in the treatment of premenstrual syndrome: systematic review. *British Medical Journal* 316:1375-1381.

Chapter 4
Weight Management and Exercise

American Yoga Association. 2001. Using yoga techniques to help relieve PMS and menopause; www.americanyogaassociation.org/onesheets/19menopause.html (3/5/01).

Baron, R. B. 1997. Treating obesity: Diet, exercise, and phen-fen. *Audio-Digest Obstetrics and Gynecology* 44(5).

Barrette, E. P. 2000. Metabolife 356 for weight loss. *Alternative Medicine Alert* 3(1):1-6.

Butts, N. K., and S. Price. 1994. Effects of a 12-week weight training program on the body composition of women over 30 years of age. *Journal of Strength Conditioning Research* 8:265-269.

Centers for Disease Control and Prevention. 2000. Prevalence of overweight and obesity among adults: United States, 1999. www.cdc.gov/nchs.

Daoust, J., and G. Daoust. 1996. *Fat Burning Nutrition.* Del Mar, Calif.: Wharton Publishing.

Davidson, M. H., et al. 1999. Weight control and risk factor reduction in obese subjects treated 2 years with Orlistat. *Journal of the American Medical Association* 281(3):235-242.

Horm, J., and K. Anderson. 1993. Who in America is trying to lose weight? *Annals of Internal Medicine* 119:672-276.

Institute of Medicine. 1995. *Weighing the Options: Criteria for Evaluating Weight-Management Programs.* Washington, D.C.: National Academy Press.

Kayman, S., W. Bruvold, and J. Stern. 1990. Maintenance and relapse after weight loss in women: Behavioral aspects. *American Journal of Clinical Nutrition* 52:800-807.

Langreth, R. 1997. Alternatives to redux still are years away. *Wall Street Journal,* September 16.

Moline, L. 1993. Pharmacological strategies for managing premenstrual syndrome. *Clinical Pharmacology* 12:181-196.

Notelovitz, M., and D. Tonnessen. 1993. *Menopause and Midlife Health.* New York: St. Martin's Press.

Ojeda, L. 1995. *Menopause without Medicine.* Alameda, Calif.: Hunter House.

O'Mathuna, D. P. 1999. Pyruvate for the treatment of obesity. *Alternative Medicine Alert* 2(3):31-33.

Pearlstein, T. B., A. Rivera-Tovar, and E. Frank. 1992. Nonmedical management of LLPDD: A preliminary report. *Journal of Psychotherapeutic Practice and Research* 1:49-55.

Prior, J. C., et al. 1997. Conditioning exercise decreases premenstrual symptoms: A prospective, controlled 6-month trial. *Fertility and Sterility* 47:402-408.

Roubenoff, R., G. E. Dallal, and P. W. F. Wilson. 1995. Predicting body fatness: The body mass index vs. estimation by bioelectrical impedance. *American Journal of Public Health* 85:726-728.

Schwarzbein, D., 1999. *The Schwarzbein Principle.* Deerfield Beach, Fla.: Health Communications, Inc.

Sjostrom, L. 1998. Randomized placebo-controlled trial of Orlistat for weight loss and prevention of weight gain in obese patients. *Lancet* 352(9123):167-173.

Women's HealthSource. 1999. Weight Control, Special Report. Mayo Foundation for Medical Education and Research. Rochester, MN, 55905; 800-430-9699.

Chapter 5
Integrative Medical Therapies

Bayne, H. M. 2000. FDA publishes new draft guidance for botanical drug products. *Herbalgram* 50:68-69.

Bienfield, H., and E. Korngold. 1991. *Between Heaven and Earth: A Guide to Chinese Medicine*. New York: Ballantine Books.

Blumenthal, M., W. R. Busse, and A. Goldberg. 1998. *The Complete German Commission E Monographs, Therapeutic Guide to Herbal Medicines*. Austin, Tex.: American Botanical Council.

Brevcort, P. 1998. The booming US botanical market: A new overview. *HerbalGram* 44:33-48.

Budeiri, D., A. Li Wan Po, and J. C. Doman. 1996. Is evening primrose oil of value in the treatment of premenstrual syndrome? *Controlled Clinical Trials* 17:60-68.

Collinge W. 1996. *The American Holistic Association Complete Guide to Alternative Medicine*. New York: Warner Books.

Fugh-Berman A. 1997. *Alternative Medicine: What Works*. Baltimore: Lippincott, Williams and Wilkins.

Garges, H. P., et al. 1998. Cardiac complications and delirium associated with valerian root withdrawal. *Journal of the American Medical Association* 280:1566-1567.

Goldberg, B. 1999. *Alternative Medicine: The Definitive Guide*. Tiburon, Calif.: Future Medicine Publishing, Inc.

Hardy, M. L. 1999. Valerian root for insomnia. *Alternative Medicine Alert* 2(8):85-88.

———. 2000. Herbs of special interest to women. *Journal of the American Pharmaceutical Association* 40:234-242.

Johnson, J. R. 1998. Premenstrual syndrome therapy. *Clinical Obstetrics and Gynecology* 41:405-421.

Khoo, S. K., C. Munro, and D. Battistutta. 1990. Evening primrose oil and treatment of premenstrual syndrome. *The Medical Journal of Australia* 153:189-192.

Kleijnen, J. 1994. Evening primrose oil: currently used in many conditions with little justification. *British Medical Journal* 309:824-825.

Ko, R. J. 1998. Adulterants in Asian patent medicines. *New England Journal of Medicine* 339:847.

Kraemer, G. R., and R. R. Kraemer. 1998. Premenstrual syndrome. Diagnosis and treatment experiences. *Journal of Women's Health* 7:893-907.

Lark, S. M. 1993. *PMS: Premenstrual Syndrome Self Help Book*. Berkeley, Calif.: Celestial Arts.

Lauritzen, C., R. D. Reuter, and R. Repges. 1997. Treatment of premenstrual tension syndrome with Vitus agnus castus: A controlled, double-blind study versus pyridoxine. *Phytomedicine* 4:183-189.

Milan, F. 2001. An overview of herbal medicine for the primary care provider: An evidence-based approach. *Primary Care Reports* 7(13):106-116.

Ondrizek, R. R. 1999. An alternative medicine study of herbal effects on the penetration of zona-free hamster oocytes and the integrity of sperm deoxyribonucleic acid. *Fertility and Sterility* 71(3):517-522.

Qi-bing, M., T. Jing-yi, and C. Bo. 1991. Advance in the pharmacological studies of radix Angelica sinensis (oliv) diels (Chinese danggui). *Chinese Medical Journal* 104:776-781.

Reichman, J. 1996. *I'm Too Young to Get Old: Health Care for Women After Forty.* New York: Times Books.

Scheidermeyer, D. 1998. Little evidence for ginseng as treatment for menopausal symptoms. *Alternative Medicine Alert* 1(7):77-78.

Schellenberg, R. 2001. Treatment for the premenstrual syndrome with agnus castus fruit extract: Prospective, randomized, placebo-controlled study. *British Medical Journal* 322:134-137.

Stevinson, C., and E. Adzard. 2001. Complimentary/alternative therapies for premenstrual syndrome: A systematic review of randomized controlled trials. *American Journal of Obstetrics and Gynecology* 185:227-235.

Tyler, V. E. 1997. The bright side of black cohosh. *Prevention* 4:76-79.

Ullman, D. 1991. *Discovering Homeopathic Medicine for the 21st Century.* Berkeley, Calif.: North Atlantic Books.

Vogler, B. K., M. H. Pittler, and E. Ernst. 1999. The efficacy of ginseng . A systematic review of randomized, clinical trials. *European Journal of Clinical Pharmacology* 55:556-575.

Wellness Letter. 2000a. Worry wort. *University of California at Berkeley Wellness Letter* 16(8):7.

Wellness Letter. 2000b. The herb with a thousand faces. *University of California at Berkeley Wellness Letter* 16(10):2-3.

Women's HealthSource. 2000. Herbs and surgery don't mix. *Mayo Clinic Women's HealthSource* 4(3):8

Chapter 6
Medications That May Help

ACOG (American College of Obstetricians and Gynecologists). 2000. Premenstrual syndrome: Clinical management guidelines for obstetrician-gynecologists. *ACOG Practice Bulletin* 15:1-9.

Backstrom, T., et al., 1992. Oral contraceptives in premenstrual syndrome: A randomized comparison of triphasic and monophasic preparations. *Contraception* 17 (suppl. 20):17-19.

Barnhart, K. T., E. W. Freeman, and S. J. Sondheimer. 1995. A Clinician's Guide to the Premenstrual Syndrome. *Medical Clinics of North America* 79:1457–1473.

Brown, C. 2001. Investigational pill may also be effective for treating PMDD. *WebMDHealth*; www.webmd.com (6/13/01).

Casson, P., et al. 1990. Lasting response to ovariectomy in severe intractable premenstrual syndrome. *American Journal of Obstetrics and Gynecology* 162:99.

DiCarlo, C., et al. 1997. Hormonal treatment of premenstrual syndrome. *Cephalgia* 17(suppl. 20):17-19.

Epperson, C. N., K. L. Wisner, and B. Yamamoto. 1999 Gonadal steroids in the treatment of mood disorders. *Psychosomatic Medicine* 61(5):676-697.

Eriksson, E. 1999. Serotonin reuptake inhibitors for the treatment of premenstrual dysphoria. *International Clinics in Psychopharmacology* 14(suppl. 2):S27-33.

Eriksson, E., et al. 1995. The serotonin reuptake inhibitor paroxetine is superior to the noradrenaline reuptake inhibitor maprotiline in the treatment of premenstrual syndrome. *Neuropsychopharmacology* 12:167-176.

Facchinetti, F., et al. 1989. Naproxen sodium in the treatment of premenstrual symptoms: a placebo controlled study. *Gynecological and Obstetrical Investigation* 28:205-208.

Fava, M., et al. 1998 An open trial of oral sildenafil in antidepressant-induced sexual dysfunction *Psychotherapy and Psychosomatics* 67:328-331.

Freeman, E. W., et al. 1993. Gonadotropin-releasing hormone agonist in treatment of premenstrual symptoms with and without comorbidity of depression: a pilot study. *Journal of Clinical Psychiatry* 54(5):192-195.

Freeman, E. W., et al. 1999. Full- or half-cycle treatment of severe premenstrual syndrome with a serotonergic antidepressant. *Journal of Clinical Psychopharmacology* 19(1):3-8.

Freeman, E. W., K. Rickels, and S. J. Sondheimer. 1990. Ineffectiveness of progesterone suppository treatment for premenstrual syndrome. *Journal of the American Medical Association* 264:349-356.

———. 1994. Nefazodone in the treatment of premenstrual syndrome: a preliminary study. *Journal of Clinical Psychopharmacology* 14(3):180-186.

Harrison, W. M., J. Endicott, and J. Nee. 1990. Treatment of premenstrual dysphoria with alprazolam. A controlled study. *Archives of General Psychiatry* 47:270-275.

Huston, J. E., and D. L. Lanka. 2001. *Perimenopause: Changes in Women's Health After 35.* Oakland, Calif.: New Harbinger Publications.

Jermain, D. M., et al. 1999 Luteal phase sertraline treatment for premenstrual dysphoric disorder. Results of a double-blind, placebo-controlled crossover study. *Archives of Family Medicine* 8(4):328-332.

Labbate, L. A., and M. H. Pollack. 1994 Treatment of fluoxetine-induced sexual dysfunction with bupropion: A case study. *Annals of Clinical Psychiatry* 6:13-15.

Lanka, L. D., and J. Klingman. 1997. Research in progress on ongoing evaluation of the use of testosterone pellets in the treatment of recalcitrant menstrual migraines. Lecture at Kaiser Foundation Hospital, Walnut Creek, Calif.

Leather, A. T., et al. 1999 The treatment of severe premenstrual syndrome with goserelin with and without "add-back" estrogen therapy: A placebo-controlled trial. *Gynecological Endocrinology* 13(1):48-55.

Leventhal, J. 1996. Premenstrual dysphoric disorder. Lecture given 15 October to the women's health department, Kaiser, Walnut Creek, Calif.

Leventhal, J. 1997. Libido and menopause. Lecture given 1 April to the women's health department, Kaiser, Walnut Creek, Calif.

Medical Economics Company. 2000. *Physicians Desk Reference*, 55th ed. Montvale, N.J.: Medical Economics Company.

Modell, J. G., et al. 1997. Comparative sexual side effects of bupropion, fluoxetine, paroxetine, and sertraline: Pharmacoepidemiology and drug utilization. *Clinical Pharmacology and Therapeutics* 61(4):476-487.

Moline, M. L., and S. M. Zendell. 1997. Evaluating and managing premenstrual syndrome. *Medscape Women's Health* 2:3.

Mortola, J. F. 1992. Issues in the diagnosis and research of premenstrual syndrome. *Clinics of Obstetrics and Gynecology* 35:587–598.

_____. 1994. A risk-benefit appraisal of drugs used in the management of premenstrual syndrome. *Drug Safety* 10:160-169.

_____. 1997. From GnRH to SSRIs and beyond: Weighing the options for drug therapy in premenstrual syndrome. *Medscape Women's Health* 2:3.

Mortola, J. F., and F. A. Moossazadeh. 1991. A randomized trial of fluoxetine and imiprimine in the treatment of premenstrual syndrome. *Proceedings of the 38th Annual Meeting of the Society for Gynecologic Investigation, March 20-23, San Antonio, Texas:* Gynecologic Investigation, Inc.

Nicolai, T. F., G. M. Mulligan, and R. K. Gribble. 1990. Thyroid function and treatment in premenstrual syndrome. *Journal of Clinical Endocrinology and Metabolism* 70:1108-1113.

Pallanti, S., and L. M. Koran. 1999. Citalopram and sexual side effects of selective serotonin reuptake inhibitors. *American Journal of Psychiatry* 156(5):796.

Revlin, M. E., J. C. Morrison, and G. W. Bates. 1990. *Manual of Clinical Problems in Obstetrics and Gynecology*, 3rd ed. Boston: Little Brown.

Rubinow, D. 1992. The premenstrual syndrome: New views. *Journal of the American Medical Association* 268:1908.

Schmidt, P. J., G. N. Grover, and D. R. Rubinow. 1993. Alprazolam in the treatment of premenstrual syndrome. A double-blind, placebo-controlled trial. *Archives of General Psychiatry* 50:467-473.

Silverstein, S. D. 1992. Advances in understanding the pathophysiology of headaches. *Neurology* 42(2):6-10.

Singh, B. B., et al. 1998. Incidence of premenstrual syndrome and remedy usage: A national probability sample study. *Alternative Therapeutic Health Medicine* 4(3):75-79.

Smith, S., and I. Schiff. 1993. *Modern Management of Premenstrual Syndrome*. New York: Norton.

Su, T. P., P. J. Schmidt, and M. A. Danaceau. 1997. Fluoxetine in the treatment of premenstrual dysphoria. *Neuropsychopharmacology* 16:346-356.

Thys-Jacobs, S. 1994. Vitamin D and calcium in menstrual migraine. *Headache* 34:544-546.

Wang, M., L. Hammarback, and T. Backstrom. 1995. Treatment of premenstrual syndrome by spironolactone: A double-blind, placebo-controlled study. *Acta Obstetrics and Gynecology of Scandinavia* 74:803-808.

Warshaw, M. G., and M. B. Keller. 1996. The relationship between fluoxetine use and suicidal behavior in 654 subjects with anxiety disorders. *Journal of Clinical Psychiatry* 57(4):158-166.

Yonkers, K. A. et al. 1997. Symptomatic improvement of premenstrual dysphoric disorder with sertraline treatment. A randomized controlled trial. Sertraline Premenstrual Dysphoric Disorder Collaborative Study Group. *Journal of the American Medical Association* 278:983-988.

Chapter 7
Stress: A PMDD Culprit

Benson, H., and E. Stuart. 1993. *The Wellness Book: The Comprehensive Guide to Maintaining and Treating Stress-Related Illness*. New York: Fireside.

Breathnach, S. B. 1995. *Simple Abundance: A Daybook of Comfort and Joy*. New York: Warner Books.

Harvard Women's Health Watch. 1999. Gender and stress. *Harvard Women's Health Watch* 7(2):1.

Hauri, P., and S. Linde. 1990. *No More Sleepless Nights*. New York: John Wiley and Sons.

Huston, J. E., and L. D. Lanka. 2001. *Perimenopause: Changes in Women's Health After 35*. Oakland, Calif.: New Harbinger Publications.

Jacobsen, E. 1974. *Progressive Relaxation*. Chicago: The University of Chicago Press.

Kiecolt-Glaser, J. 1996. The negative influence of stress on the immune system. Presentation at the annual meeting of The International Society of Neuroimmunomodulation.

Kiecolt-Glaser, J., and R. Glaser. 1991. Stress and immune function in humans. In *Psychoneuroimmunology*, 2nd ed., edited by, R. Ader, D. L. Felten, and N. Cohen. San Diego, Calif.: Academic Press.

Kobasa, S., S. Maddi, and S. Kahn. 1982. Hardiness and health: A prospective study. *Journal of Personality and Social Psychology* 42:168-177.

Landau, C., M. Cyre, and A. Moutlon. 1994. *The Complete Book of Menopause: Every Woman's Guide to Good Health*. New York: G. P. Putnam's Sons.

McKay M, M. Davis, and P. Fanning. 1997. *Thoughts and Feelings: Taking Control of Your Moods and Your Life*. Oakland, Calif.: New Harbinger Publications.

Moyers, B. 1993. *Healing and the Mind*. New York: Bantam Doubleday Dell.

Notelovitz, M., and D. Tonnessen. 1993. *Menopause and Midlife Health*. New York: St. Martin's Press.

Wilde, L. 1997. Humor: Rx for healing, health, and happiness. Lecture given 22 April at the Rogue Valley Medical Center, Medford, Oregon.

Chapter 8
Cognitive Behavioral Therapy

Beck, A. T. 1963. Thinking and depression. 1. Idiosyncratic content and cognitive distortions. *Archives of General Psychiatry* 9:324-333.

———. 1967. *Depression: Clinical, Experimental, and Theoretical Aspects*. New York: Hoeber. (Republished in 1972 as *Depression: Causes and Treatment*. Philadelphia: University of Pennsylvania Press.)

Beck, A.T., et al. 1979. *Cognitive Therapy of Depression*. New York: Guilford Press.

Davis, L., and K. A. Yonkers. 1997. Diagnosis and treatment of premenstrual dysphoric disorder. *International Journal of Psychiatry in Clinical Practice* 1(3):149-156.

Ellis, A. 1962. *Reason and Emotion in Psychotherapy*. Secaucus, N.J.: Citadel.

———. 1984. Foreword. In W. Bryden, *Rational-Emotive Therapy: Fundamentals and Innovations* London: Croom Helm.

———. 1999. *How to Make Yourself Happy and Remarkably Less Disturbable*. San Luis Obispo, Calif.: Impact Publishers.

Ellis, A., and M. E. Bernard. 1986. What is rational-emotive therapy (RET)? In *Handbook of Rational-Emotive Therapy*, vol. 2, edited by A. Ellis and R. Grieger. New York: Springer.

Ellis, A., and R. Grieger, eds. 1977. *Handbook of Rational-Emotive Therapy* Vol. 1. New York: Springer.

Ellis, A., and R. A Harper. 1979. *A New Guide to Rational Living*. (Revised.) Englewood Cliffs, N.J.: Prentice-Hall.

Kirkby, R. J. 1994. Changes in premenstrual symptoms and irrational thinking following cognitive behavioral coping skill training. *Journal of Consulting Clinical Psychology* 62:1026-1032.

Koons, S. R. 1999. Cognitive-behavioral symptom management of premenstrual dysphoric disorder: A multi-element design with replications. *Dissertation Abstracts International: Section B: The Sciences and Engineering* 60(5B):2346.

Chapter 9
Mood Disorders and PMDD

APA (American Psychiatric Association). 1994. *Diagnostic and Statistical Manual of Mental Disorders,* 4th ed. Washington, D.C.: APA.

Bailey, J. W., and L. S. Cohen. 1999. Prevalence of mood and anxiety disorders in women who seek treatment for premenstrual syndrome. *Journal of Women's Health and Gender Based Medicine* 8(9):1181-1184.

Flett, G., K. Vredenburg, and L. Krames. 1997. The continuity of depression in clinical and nonclinical samples. *Psychological Bulletin* 121:395-416.

Lang, P. 1967. Fear reduction and fear behavior. In *Research in Psychotherapy*, edited by J. Schlein. Washington, D.C.: American Psychological Association.

Judd, L., et al. 1996. Functional impairment associated with subsyndromal depression. *American Journal of Psychiatry* 153:1411-1417.

Monroe, S., et al. 1999. Life events and depression in adolescence. Relationship loss as a prospective risk factor for first onset of major depressive disorder. *Journal of Abnormal Psychology* 108:606-614.

Rachman, S. J. 1978. *Fear and Courage.* New York: Freeman.

Chapter 10
Tying it All Together

Barbach, L. 1993. *The Pause: Positive Approaches to Menopause*. New York: Signet Books.

James E. Huston, M.D., specialized in obstetrics and gynecology before his retirement. He now lectures across the country on women's health concerns, and is the co-author of *Perimenopause: Changes in Women's Health after 35*. He lives in Medford, Oregon.

Lani C. Fujitsubo, Ph.D. is a clinical psychologist in private practice in southern Oregon. She is also the Associate Professor of Psychology, Southern Oregon University; and the Director of Testing at Southern Oregon University.

Some Other
New Harbinger Titles

The Deepest Blue, Item DPSB $13.95

The 50 Best Ways to Simplify Your Life, Item FWSL $11.95

Brave New You, Item BVNY $13.95

Loving Your Teenage Daughter, Item LYTD $14.95

The Hidden Feelings of Motherhood, Item HFM $14.95

The Woman's Book of Sleep, Item WBS $14.95

Pregnancy Stories, Item PS $14.95

The Women's Guide to Total Self-Esteem, Item WGTS $13.95

Thinking Pregnant, Item TKPG $13.95

The Conscious Bride, Item CB $12.95

Juicy Tomatoes, Item JTOM $13.95

Facing 30, Item F30 $12.95

The Money Mystique, Item MYST $13.95

High on Stress, Item HOS $13.95

Perimenopause, 2nd edition, Item PER2 $16.95

The Infertility Survival Guide, Item ISG $16.95

After the Breakup, ATB $13.95

Claiming Your Creative Self, Item CYCS $15.95

The Self-Nourishment Companion, Item SNC $10.95

Serenity to Go, Item STG $12.95

Spiritual Housecleaning, Item SH $12.95

Goodbye Good Girl, Item GGG $12.95

Under Her Wing, Item WING $13.95

Goodbye Mother, Hello Woman, Item GOOD $14.95

Call **toll free, 1-800-748-6273,** or log on to our online bookstore at **www.newharbinger.com** to order. Have your Visa or Mastercard number ready. Or send a check for the titles you want to New Harbinger Publications, Inc., 5674 Shattuck Ave., Oakland, CA 94609. Include $4.50 for the first book and 75¢ for each additional book, to cover shipping and handling. (California residents please include appropriate sales tax.) Allow two to five weeks for delivery.

Prices subject to change without notice.